THE CASE REPORTS AND AUTOPSY
RECORDS OF AMBROISE PARÉ

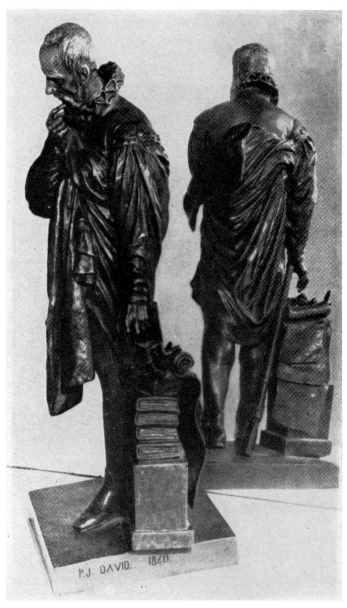

PARÉ'S STATUE BY DAVID D'ANGERS
(Courtesy Mr. E. Weil, London)

THE CASE REPORTS
AND AUTOPSY RECORDS
OF AMBROISE PARÉ

Compiled and Edited by

WALLACE B. HAMBY, M.D., F.A.C.S.

Department of Neurological Surgery
Cleveland Clinic
Cleveland, Ohio

Translated from

J. P. MALGAIGNE'S

"Oeuvres Completes d'Ambroise Paré"
Paris, 1840

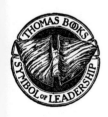

CHARLES C THOMAS • PUBLISHER
Springfield • Illinois • U.S.A.

CHARLES C THOMAS · PUBLISHER

BANNERSTONE HOUSE

301-327 EAST LAWRENCE AVENUE, SPRINGFIELD, ILLINOIS, U.S.A.

Published simultaneously in the British Commonwealth of Nations by

BLACKWELL SCIENTIFIC PUBLICATIONS, LTD., OXFORD, ENGLAND

Published simultaneously in Canada by

THE RYERSON PRESS, TORONTO

© *1960, by* CHARLES C THOMAS · PUBLISHER

Library of Congress Catalog Card Number: 60-12663

With THOMAS BOOKS *careful attention is given to all details of
manufacturing and design. It is the Publisher's desire to present books
that are satisfactory as to their physical qualities and artistic possibilities
and appropriate for their particular use.* THOMAS BOOKS *will be true
to those laws of quality that assure a good name and good will.*

Printed in the United States of America

This little book is affectionately dedicated to my long-time (1934-1960) Colleagues of the University of Buffalo, School of Medicine, The Buffalo General Hospital and the local Profession, who generously favored me with all the help and the honors at their command.

Introduction

SEVERAL unusual lines of influence converged in the 16th Century to make the life and writings of Ambroise Paré of special interest to his successors. He happened to be born at the onset and to live practically to the end of one of the most stirring centuries of French history. The medieval age had slipped away and Europeans became aware that the expected end of the world was at least a little deferred. Explorers had shown the horizons to be wider than anticipated and that life need not necessarily be constrained in the traditional limits, but could expand in exciting directions. A stirring and leavening developed in all phases of experience, moving, cracking through and sometimes shattering the comfortable encompassing limits set by Authority.

Among the human activities neatly formulated and safely bound to the status quo by the accumulated treasury of the knowledge of centuries was French Medicine and Surgery. No less rigidly than the Church had its devotees enclosed themselves within a cage of authority and protection. It had its own language, Latin, that must be mastered before its candidates could enter the hallowed precincts and in this language alone could they communicate. And so communicating, they were free-of-tongue with the whole civilized world, privy to secrets of their order anywhere. Within the walls of this medieval cosmos were delineated the boundaries for the various classes of the crowded but orderly anthill. The Physicians, Patricians of the lot, were governed by and obeyed the legally appointed heirarchy of the Faculty of Medicine. These men walked proudly in their long robes, their white hands withdrawn cleanly into their sleeves, unsullied by contact with their patients. Surgery was the duty and privilege of a second order, Surgeons of the College of St. Côme, whose graduates wore the Long Robe and were licensed to practice. The rules of this group were as restricting and protective as were those of the Physicians, and their practitioners, looking always upward at the Physicians, aspired to their arid heights and took on their coloring. One by one they abandoned tasks that were physically difficult, dangerous and dirty, and these were many in the days of surgery before anesthesia and asepsis. Even though life was cheap and overly plentiful in the teeming confines of the crowded walled cities, some manual work must be done in surgery; this was pushed upon a rough, uncouth and uneducated group of servitors, the barbers. Some of these, dextrous with the razor and its gradually evolved, specialized forms of complementary instruments, became sufficiently accomplished to be called Barber-Surgeons. A few of these, overburdened with the bulk of work grown too great for small numbers, maintained and even trained apprentices. Some of these, dissatisfied at remaining at an assistant's level, launched into practices of their own, rather than keeping their places. Their masters were careful that they did not learn too much, and the surgeons took care that teaching and writing of real surgery remained in Latin, which effectively kept these worthies at their heels. Finally the Barber-Surgeons set up their own corporation, with Saints Damien and Cosmo as their patrons. A license was required of those becoming Masters.

Into this orderly, inter-meshing Parisian mechanism

strode Ambroise Paré about 1533. Son, probably, of a
Barber-Surgeon of Laval, certainly brother of one of
Vitré and having one for a brother-in-law in Paris, he had
the background and knew the limits of his craft. After his
apprenticeship, being uncertain of his training and too poor
to pay the fees for examination for license to practice, he
served as "house-officer" for three or four years in the
Hôtel-Dieu. This was Paris' only charity hospital at the
front door of and, indeed, partly overlapping the west
facade of Nôtre-Dame itself. Here he developed the senti-
ments for the highest ideals of surgery, and blessed with
adequate dexterity and a brain capable of assimilating the
mysteries of his betters, he was restrained only by lack of
communication to existence on an inferior level.

Shrugging off and side-stepping the apparent inevitable,
he cast his lot in the field of military surgery, where brief,
humane contact with suffering patients brought its own
reward. His ascent was swift, but he yearned to improve the
abilities of those who, like himself, must care for people.
On his first journey to Turin (Torino, Italy) in 1537, he
made pioneer observations that even Professor Sylvius
urged him to write. What if the French language at the
time was merely a conglomeration of local patois, was not
Ronsard at François' Court presently campaigning for its
standardization? And another seam appeared in the pro-
fessional strait jacket; a Barber-Surgeon friend, Étienne
de la Rivière, had helped a Physician, Charles Estienne,
write an anatomical treatice and his right to recognition in
print was being considered in the courts. Shortly after the
case was decided in his favor, Paré's little book of sixty-four
pages and twenty-three wood-cut illustrations on *The
Method of Treating Wounds Made by Firearms,* etc. appeared in 1545.

The sequel is sketchily known to every modern medical

student. With his tremendous energy, skill and charm, Paré moved on to a tremendous practice, wrote a series of eagerly awaited books and moved up the surgical ladder to become Surgeon to four and finally Premier-Surgeon and Councilor to the last two Valois Kings. He was admitted to the august membership of the Royal College of Surgeons, although he never learned Latin. He lived through the Religious Wars that tore the country apart and was respected by both sides for his impartial attitude as a man who had his hands entirely full minding his own business. He died at the age of eighty and was buried around the corner from his houses in the little Church he had attended since opening his "shop" in the city.

Before the Case Reports is included a "Chronology of Ambroise Paré and his Era" compiled to orient the reader on the flow of personal, local and a few noteworthy foreign events occurring during the eighty years of Paré's life. This tabulation has been gathered over the years from various sources and no doubt contains minor errors in time. Some of the dates mentioned by Paré himself were corrected by Malgaigne from general history. Another source of confusion in dates relates to the shift of New Year's Day from Easter to January 1st, which was accomplished in 1566, according to Doe (p. 52).

Paré wrote voluminously and in the 350 years since his death, much has been written about him. Yet for one who does not read French, it will be difficult to find anything of his to read that is not colored by the Elizabethan language of Th. Johnson, who translated his *Oeuvres* into English in 1634.

In 1840 Malgaigne reprinted the Fifth Edition of Paré's *Oeuvres* in modern French, with an elaborate analysis and critique of his surgery. This is the most valuable, easily obtainable source of the old Master's work; his original books have gradually been collected by libraries, making chance escapees entirely too expensive for the average man. Charmingly told stories of his life and times by Paget, Singer and Packard are out of print.

Janet Doe's 1937 *Bibliography of the Works of Ambroise Paré* contains many interesting facts of his life, his books and the men who printed them for him.

Geoffrey Keynes last reprinted his *Apologie and Treatise* in 1952, with selections of other extracts from Johnson's translation.

Charming as it is, Johnson's Elizabethan English gives the modern reader a little distorted flavor to the old Frenchman and his work. He has even become considered "quaint," I fear in the same use of the term reserved for anti-macassars and bogus antiques of other sorts. The word applied to Paré is as insulting as it would be in the case of George Washington or Benjamin Franklin.

It has seemed that a modern English translation of Paré would be worthwhile, but as Miss Doe pointed out to me, the bulk of his surgical writing is so long outdated and so heavily weighted with Renaissance concepts of pathophysiology, it would be of little value to anyone. His case reports are another matter, as it was from his own observations that he was shrewd enough to draw his conclusions for treatment. Some of these constitute the most interesting parts of the reprints of Johnson's translation.

In search of his original accounts of personal experiences I have gone through Malgaigne's reprint of the Fifth Edition of Paré's *Oeuvres* and have translated each of his personal case reports and his autopsy reports. It is amazing to see how much he learned of his predecessors' writings from obtainable French translations, and how many of their case reports he included in his books. These have not been included here, nor have been those he reported having heard from his contemporaries. Unfortunately, my knowledge of French is a poor tool for the task undertaken and Sixteenth Century French is difficult for even a modern Frenchman. I believe the facts are fairly accurately reported, however, even if the style leaves much to be desired. My own translations have been checked by Madame Jeanne Powel, a French expert of Buffalo, to avoid gross errors and I here acknowledge my great debt to her.

Each case report has been given an explanatory title. A page reference to Malgaigne has been put in parentheses beside each case heading to permit the reader to find the original text for each. Footnotes concerning facts relative to persons, places and events have been put on the text pages and designated by identifying numerals that follow the item through subsequent pages. In the index, the page carrying the explanatory foot-note is italicized. In the index, names of Physicians, Surgeons and Barber-Surgeons are identified by asterisks.

The arrangement of the Reports has not been altered, which may make them appear somewhat jumbled to one who reads continuously, but the index permits selection of associated topics. Paré included parenthetical remarks in his text and these have been indicated. Explanatory remarks by the editor have been designated by a terminal "—Ed." notation.

Some of the reports appear in more than one place, and are so presented, since each version was written to emphasize certain features of the case. This is particularly pertinent in the presentations in the last section, *"The Apology and Treatise Containing the Trips Made in Divers Places."* This was the last publication by Paré in his lifetime and appeared in the Fourth Edition of his *Oeuvres*, in 1585. Since this little book was both a defense of his individual surgical discoveries and a valuable historical account of his military surgery, it is probably the best known of all his writings. It has been reprinted, usually from Johnson's translation, several times in English.

W. B. H.

Professional Chronology of Ambroise Paré

1510   Paré born at Bourg-Hersent, suburb of Laval, France

1523   Paré apprenticed to Vialot, Barber-Surgeon, Vitre (tradition)

1531   Barber-Surgeon apprenticeship in Paris (tradition)

1533   Started service as "compagnon-chirurgien," Hôtel-Dieu, Paris

1535   Finished service at Hôtel-Dieu, practice as Barber-Surgeon

1537   To Turin, Italy, as Surgeon of duc de Montejan

1538   Death of Montejan, Paré returned to Paris

1541   Licensed as Master Barber-Surgeon

      June 30   Married to Jeanne Mazelin, Church of St. André-des-Arts

1542   To siege of Perpignan with duc de Rohan, return in month

1543   To Maroilles with de Rohan, then to Landerneau with de Rohan and de Laval; repulse of English; return to Paris

1544   To Landrecies with de Rohan

1545 Aug.   Publication book on Gunshot Wounds
                 (*La Methode de Traicter les Playes
                 Faictes par Hacquebutes, etc.*) dedicated
                 to de Rohan

     Aug.   To Boulogne with de Rohan; wound of
                 François de Guise

1547   Dutch edition of "Gunshot Wounds"
                 book

1549   Publication of Paré's Anatomy (*Briefve
                 Collection de l'Administration Anato-
                 mique, etc.*) dedicated to de Rohan

1550   Paré to Boulogne; Publication 2nd. ed.
                 of Anatomy

1552 Mar.   Publication 2nd. ed. "Gunshot Wounds"
                 dedication to Henri II

     Apr.   Paré with de Rohan in King's army, to
                 Toul, Nancy, Metz, Verdun

     July   Capture of Damvilliers, Paré first used
                 ligatures in amputation

     Aug.   To Château le Comte with King of Na-
                 varre

     Aug.   To Reims; appointment as King's Sur-
                 geon-in-Ordinary

     Oct.   Assault on Metz by Emperor, defense
                 by de Guise

     Dec.   Paré to Metz to treat defenders

     Dec. 26   Siege abandoned by Emperor

1553 Jan.   Paré back to Paris via Verdun

     June 30   Fall of Theroüenne; Paré with defense
                 to Hesdin

     July 17   Fall of Hesdin; capture of Paré; treat-
                 ment M. de Vaudeville, liberation, re-
                 turn to Paris

1554	Aug. 18	Petition by Paré to College of Surgeons for examination
	Aug. 27	Formal examination at Hôtel-Dieu
	Dec. 17	Admission to College of Surgeons as Master Surgeon
1557	Aug. 10	Battle of St. Quentin, Paré at La Fère to treat wounded
1558	Apr.	Paré to camp at Dourlan; return to Paris
1559	June 29	Tournament injury of Henri II; treated by Paré and Vesalius
	July 10	Death of Henri II, autopsy and embalmment by Paré. François II, 15 yr. old King of France
1560	Dec. 5	Death of François II, middle ear infection; autopsy and embalmment by Paré. Charles IX, 10 yr. old King of France
1561	Apr.	Publication of Paré's *Anatomie Universelle du Corps Humain,* dedicated to King of Navarre
	May 4	Compound fracture Paré's left ankle
	Sept.	Paré walking without a limp
1562	Jan. 1	Appointment as Premier Surgeon and Valet-de-Chambre by Charles IX
	Feb. 28	Publication Paré's "Head Injuries" (*La Méthode Curative des Playes, & Fractures de la Teste humaine, etc.*), dedicated to King's Premier Physician, Chapelain
	May	To Bourges with the King
	Oct. 26	Fall of Rouen, injury of King of Navarre, died despite Paré
	Dec. 19	Battle of Dreux; Paré treated wounded
1563	July	Paré at Le Havre, French vs English

1564 Jan.   Paré started with Court on 2 yr. tour
                 of France

      Feb. 3   Publication Paré's Ten Books of Sur-
                 gery (*Dix Livres de la Chirurgie, etc.*),
                 first account of use of ligatures in ampu-
                 tations. Study of plague at Lyon; to
                 Montpellier for winter

1565 Jan.   Paré bitten by snake at Montpellier

      Apr.   Arrival at Bayonne for 3 months; Paré
                 to Biarritz; via Bordeaux, Blois & Orlé-
                 ans to Paris
                 Treatment King's median nerve, injured
                 in bleeding accident

1566 Jan.   To Moulins with Court

1567   Paré's attempt to unite Surgeons under
                 King's Premier Surgeon; blocked by
                 Faculty of Medicine

      Nov. 10   Battle of St. Denis; spinal pistol wound
                 of Constable Montmorency; treatment
                 useless

1568   Publication Paré's book on Plague
                 (*Traicte de la Peste, de la Petite Verolle
                 & Rougeolle*, etc.), dedicated to Queen-
                 Mother's Premier Physician, Castellan

1569 Oct. 3   Battle of Moncontour, Paré at Plessis-
                 les-Tours treating wounded- Paré to
                 Flanders for 2 mo. to treat Marquise
                 d'Auret; visit to Brussels, Antwerp &
                 Ghent; return to Paris

1572 Mar.   Publication Paré's Five Books of Sur-
                 gery (*Cinq Livres de Chirurgie*, etc.),
                 dedicated to King Charles IX

      Aug. 24   St. Bartholomew's Day Massacre of

		Paris Huguenots; Paré kept in Louvre by King
1573		Publication Paré's Two Books of Surgery (*Deux Livres de Chirurgie*, etc.), dedicated to duc d'Uzés
	Nov. 4	Death of Paré's wife, Jeanne Mazelin, aged 53
1574	Jan. 18	Second marriage with Jacqueline Rousselet
	May 30	Death Charles IX, of tuberculosis; autopsy and embalmment by Paré Coronation King Henri III; Paré appointed Premier-Surgeon, Councilor and Valet-de-Chambre
1575	Jan.	Paré to Nancy with Marc Miron to treat duchesse de Lorraine; visit with Nicholas Picart, fracture surgeon
	Apr.	Publication Paré's Works (*Les Oeuvres de M. Ambroise Paré*, etc.), dedicated to the King
1579	Feb.	Publication 2nd. ed. Paré's *Oeuvres*
1580		Paré on Plague Commission; reissue of *Book on the Plague* of 1568
1582	Jan.	Publication of 3rd., Latin ed. of Paré's *Oeuvres* by Jacques Guillemeau, Paré's pupil
	Mar.	Publication of Paré's Book on Mummy, etc. (*Discours d'Ambroise Paré, etc., De la Mumie, de la Licorne, des Venins, et de la Peste*, etc.), dedicated to M. des Ursins
1583	Dec. 10	Still in practice, supervised amputation by assistant Poullet

1585   Publication of 4th ed. of Paré's *Oeuvres*,
                       containing the "Apology & Treatise and
                       the Journeys in Divers Places"
1589   Paré preparing 5th ed. of his *Oeuvres*
                       which appeared in 1598
1590   July   Paris under siege; Paré's plea to Head
                       of League for peace
       Dec. 20   Eve of St. Thomas; death at age 80 in
                       his house of The Three Moors, rue de
                       l'Hirondelle, of Ambroise Paré, Pre-
                       mier Surgeon, Councilor and Valet-de-
                       Chambre of the King
       Dec. 22   Burial of Paré in his church, St. André-
                       des-Arts "at the foot of the nave, near
                       the tower"

THE CASE REPORTS AND AUTOPSY
RECORDS OF AMBROISE PARÉ

The Case Reports and Autopsy Records of Ambroise Paré

Suffocation by Gluttony (MI,27)

If it is a morsal of bread or meat (lodged in the throat—Ed.) one must do as I did to one of the servants of Henry Hazard, Master Tailor of Suits, living on St. Michel's Bridge.[1] The history follows:

Six servants planned a good dinner and each contributed one liard to buy some tripe. An eating contest developed; one took a morsal of big breach gut; having put it in his mouth, it annoyed him that it was not in his stomach. He tried to swallow it without chewing. The morsal remained in his throat and could not pass, which gave him very great difficulty in breathing and he fell like an epileptic, blood spurting from his mouth, nose and ears, his face all livid and black, so they feared the poor glutton would die of this morsal of tripe. I was hurriedly brought and seeking the cause of his trouble, made them lift him on a bench chair. I took a leek and, having them remove the head and peel it,

[1] St. Michel's Bridge (Pont St. Michel), built by King Charles V (1378-1387), connected the left bank of the Seine with the street running past the Palais and the St. Chapelle. At its southern (left bank) end it led into the Place St. Michel, around which Paré lived most of his life. His nearest communication with the Isle, Paré must have crossed it innumerable times. In the 16th century it was lined on both sides with tall houses, later razed. Its counterpart on the northern end of the island was the Pont-au-Change (q.v.), guarded by the huge Châtelet. (See also 90 & 91)

3

I opened his mouth with a speculum, thrust the leek quite hard, deep into the throat and struck him with a hand between the shoulders so the morsel fell into the stomach. Being out of danger, he promptly threw his eyes on the platter where the tripes had been and began to cry out against his companions that they had eaten without him, saying they should return his money. Then Master Henry, his master, seeing that instead of thanking God for having been removed from the peril of suffocation and death, on the contrary he cried for the tripe, at once paid him his wages and discharged him saying, "Goodbye, Glutton." Since then, among his fellow Tailors of the City he was always called Glutton, because of which he returned to his own country, which is not a great loss to Paris.

Foreign Bodies in the Penis   (MI,28)

Foreign bodies can enter the penis; these are some I have seen. One day I put a little lead sound as long as a finger into the penis of a great Seigneur, for some indisposition he had. Three hours later it had entered almost to the end and if I had not seen the very tip of it, I believe it would have entered the bladder. I recovery it with great difficulty, pressing and working it carefully to the tip of the penis.

If one does not wish to believe that the bladder draws foreign bodies into itself, I could refer him to Colot,[2] who

---

[2] Colot (also spelled Collo by Paré), a famous family of lithotomists. Laurent Colot was a physician of Trainel, near Troyes. Having learned lithotomy from Marianus Sanctus, he was called to Paris in 1556 by Henri II, who appointed him Surgeon-in-Ordinary and Lithotomist to the Hôtel-Dieu. This post passed to his sons Jean and Franco who also became famous in the field. Laurent was Surgeon also to Kings François II and Charles IX. (See also 112)

found in a man named Tire-vit, a needle enveloped in a stone which he had removed from him, which he gave me and which I regard with admiration. This needle had been attached by Tire-vit to the end of a small wand which he put into his penis to push back a little stone which had entered the urethra. The needle had separated from the wand and the bladder had drawn it in and in the passage of time it was enveloped in stony matter. (see also pg. 112—Ed.)

Quartan Fever (MI,95)

The valet of young M. de Lausa, told me of a French gentleman, in Poland, having the quartan fever (malaria—Ed.). Walking along the Vistula River at the onset of his attack, he was pushed by a laughing friend into the river. Although he could swim, as was known to him who pushed him, he was so terrified that he has never since had the fever.

At the Camp at Amiens[3] (1558—Ed.), King Henri commanded me to go to Dourlan[4] to treat several captains

---

[3] Capital of Picardy, 131 Km. northeast of Paris, Amiens has been an important city since the Roman days of the 4th century. Damaged in the war of 1914-1918, it was devastated between 1940 and 1944 by bombing. Fortunately its beautiful gothic Cathedral, built between 1220 and 1247, was spared in the last holocost, and the surrounding reconstruction permits better visualization than it enjoyed before.

Paré must have visited Amiens several times on his army journeys and mentioned particularly being here with King Henri II in 1558. The King sent him on to the Army camp at Dourlan to treat the wounded. (See also 138-141-180)

[4] Dourlan (now Doullens), a village 30 Km. north of Amiens. In Paré's time a huge fortified castle stood here. The fortifications were demolished in 1867; the château remains on a hillside above the town. Paré was here in June of 1553 and in April of 1558. The latter visit

and soldiers wounded by the Spaniards who fired on them in a sortie from the town. Captain St. Aubin, as valiant a gentleman as any in France, lived near Amiens and had the quartan fever. Nevertheless, at the onset of his attack, leaving his bed and mounting his horse to command his company, he was wounded by a harquebus shot in the neck. He had such terror of death that at the moment he lost his fever, and afterward recovered from his wound and is still living. (See also pg. 180—Ed.)

A gascon in this city, lodged at the house of Agrippa on the rue Pavée, sick of a high fever, fell into a frenzy. At night he hurled himself from the window of the second floor to the pavement, injuring himself in several parts of his body. I was called to treat him and, immediately as he was put in bed, he became rational, lost his frenzy and was cured.

Pathologic Emotions   (MI,99)

An honored gentleman brought his wife to this city to get the advice of Messrs. le Grand,[5] Duret,[6] and myself, to

---

was made on the King's order to treat the wounded in the camp. Dysentery broke out and Paré did autopsies to learn the mechanism of the intestinal hemorrhages. He instituted sanitary precautions to control the epidemic. (See also 138 & 141).

[5] Nicolle le Grand, famous physician of Kings Henri II, François II, Charles IX and Henri III. He was Regent of the Paris Faculty of Medicine (LePaulmier 191).

[6] Loys Duret, born 1527, graduated in Medicine at Paris Sept. 12, 1552, was Physician-in-Ordinary to Kings Charles IX and Henri III and Professor at the College of France in 1586. Henri III attended the wedding of Duret's daughter Catherine to Arnould de l'Isle in 1588, appearing at the Church and the reception, giving the young couple all the gold and silver vessels used, valued at 40,000 livres. Duret died the following year. His son Jean became a skillful physician.

find why she wept and laughed without reason, and no one could cure her. We treated her with many remedies but could accomplish little; finally he took her away in the same state she had come.

Obsession of Poisoning (MI,99)

The Curé of Montlhéry took the notion that he had been poisoned. He came to this city and called Messrs. Houllier[7] and Sylvius,[8] famous Physicians, and myself. He complained of severe pains in all his limbs, telling us he knew he was poisoned. After being well examined, he went away while we concluded (seeing him with this firm opinion and as he had already called other Physicians who had treated him without benefit) that we should humor him by giving him some syrup of violet, of which he should take three spoonful two hours before eating for a period of nine days, assuring him it would cure him. Then he was very glad and he wished to have our prescription in writing. This was refused, for in such a case, that would be of no

---

[7] Jacques Houllier, also spelled by Paré—Holier, Hollier and Houlier. He was mentioned as a consultant seven times by Paré, who described him as a "Regent Physician of the Faculty of Medicine," "a famous physician," "a learned doctor," etc. Unfortunately, I have found nothing more about him than Paré offered.

[8] "Sylvius" was the name used by Dr. Jacques du Bois. He was born in 1478 at Louvilly, near Amiens, studied anatomy under Tagault and graduated in Medicine at Montpellier. Coming to Paris he became a Professor of the Faculty and had an extensive practice. Vesalius came to Paris to study anatomy with him and was rather disappointed to find him a traditional Galenist rather than an investigator. The two later quarrelled violently over Vesalius' writings. Sylvius used young Paré as a prosecutor and encouraged him to publish his discoveries in the treatment of gunshot wounds. He died on January 13, 1555 and was buried in the Cemetery for Poor Scholars.

benefit to him. The Apothecary gave him the syrup in a vial, praising it as an excellent drug against his poison. And just as he took the idea of having been poisoned, so did he of being dis-empoisoned by this syrup. A month later he returned to us to thank us for our assistance; and he was gay and happy, no longer in pain, and gave each of us a livre.

Obsession of Brain Disease   (MI,100)

A gentleman otherwise well, had the idea his brain was rotten. He went to the King, begging him to command M. le Grand, Physician, M. Pigray,[9] King's Surgeon-in-Ordinary and myself, to open his head, remove his diseased brain and replace it with another. We did many things to him but it was impossible for us to restore his brain.

Delusion of Syphilis   (MI,100)

I saw a man convinced that he had syphilis and could not by any argument convince him he did not have it. He told me that if I did not treat him as he desired he would go to someone else to rub him (with mercury—Ed.). Seeing him of such will, for fear he would fall into the hands of some quack who would possibly rub him in earnest, I

---

[9] Pierre Pigray was born in Paris in 1531 and lived in Paré's house as a pupil for several years. He also followed the armies and qualified as a Master in Surgery in 1564, being appointed Surgeon-in-Ordinary by Kings Charles IX, Henri III and Henri IV. He and Portail[64] were with Henri III when he was stabbed by Jacques Clement in 1588. Paré, altho Premier Surgeon, was not with the King that day, being to old to make the trip. Pigray was Dean of the College of Surgeons in 1609 and died on October 15, 1613.

agreed that he should be rubbed as one would do in treating syphilis. I took a pound of butter beaten in a lead mortar to give it the color of an ointment containing mercury. He was rubbed with the said butter and sweated on three separate days, and each day he said his pains diminished. Thus he was cured by opinion, without any offense to his body.

Imaginary Horns (MI,100)

One can speak here of having seen others who stubbornly persuaded themselves of having horns. The fantasy can not be torn from their melancholy and bizarre brains until, their eyes being covered, the forehead is scratched on each side with beef horns, so that by the painful effusion of their own blood they persuaded themselves that such horns had really been torn out by force. There are many other such histories that I omit for brevity.

Gunshot Wound of Chest (MI,102)

At the last assault of Hesdin[10] (July 17, 1553), the elder M. de Martigues[11] was shot through the chest with an

---

[10] Hesdin today is a simple Flemish village of 3500 people, 68 Km. north of Ameins. In the 16th century it was a French strong-hold with a huge castle and fort, guarding the way to Boulogne. After their repulse at Metz in 1552, the Spanish under the duc de Savoy struck the fort in July of 1553. The surprised French were unprepared, and insufficient reinforcements under François de Montmorency, the Constable's son, were sent to hold it. Paré went with them and escaped with his life when the castle fell only by disguising as a servant of M. de Martigues. Paré's account of the siege is one of the best-told tales in his "Journeys." Savoy destroyed the place as a fortress completely.

[11] Charles de Luxembourg, Vicomte de Martigues, was son of François II of Luxembourg. He participated in the defense of Metz in 1552 and

arquebus. I treated him with the Physicians and Surgeons of the late Emperor Charles[12] and those of M. the duc de Savoy,[13] who greatly desired his recovery. For this he called a consultation where we agreed that the patient would die of his wound, since the ball had passed through the lungs and since a great quantity of blood had gathered in the thorax. A Spanish imposter appeared, who undertook to cure him at the cost of his own life; which caused M. the duc de Savoy, in view of our prognosis, to place him entirely in the hands of this venerable imposter. He demanded one of Seigneur de Martigues' shirts which he tore into small strips which he placed in form of a cross (with certain words), on his wounds and permitted him to eat and drink what he would; he said he would diet for him. This he did, eating only a few prunes and drinking only beer. Despite all this, the Seigneur de Martigues died

---

was mortally wounded in the defense of Hesdin a year later. Paré treated him there. He had married Claude de Foix, widow of the Comte de Laval, an old friend of Paré.

[12] Charles V, Emperor (1500-1558), grandson of Ferdinand of Aragon and Isabella of Castile and of Emperor Maximillian I and Mary of Burgundy. Inheriting the Spanish dominions in 1516 and the Austrian and Burgundian in 1519, he was elected Emperor of Germany and the Holy Roman Empire the same year, defeating King François I for the honor. He fought François and Henri II through his entire reign over the Burgundian and Italian States, sacking Rome and capturing the Pope in 1527. Later he persecuted the Protestants in the Netherlands and banished them from Spain. A gluttonous eater, he suffered severely from gout, which impelled his abdication in 1556 in favor of his son, Philip II of Spain.

[13] Emmanuel Philibert, duc de Savoy, the "Iron-Head" (1528-1580). General under the Emperor Charles V at Metz and Hesdin, he won the battle of St. Lawrence (St. Quentin) from the French under the Constable Montmorency, August 10, 1557. After the Peace of Château Cambresis, 1559, he married Marguerite, sister of his late adversary, King Henri II of France, who was killed at a tournament held partly in celebration of the wedding.

two days later and my Spaniard disappeared, fearing hanging for the false promises he had made. I embalmed the dead body in the presence of many Physicians, Surgeons and several Gentlemen and others, and having opened it, found the lungs pierced and lacerated, and a large quantity of blood spread on the diaphragm, which was the cause of the death of the Seigneur. (See also pg. 68 and 171—Ed.)

Lupia (Wens or Ganglions) (MI,351)

This method (ligature and amputation—Ed.) was used by M. Laurent Colot, Surgeon-in-Ordinary of the King and myself in the presence of M. de Violaines,[14] Doctor Regent of the Faculty of Medicine of Paris, greatly esteemed among learned people, on Martial Colart, Provost of Barbonne, living two leagues from Sedan. He had such a tumor the size of a man's head hanging behind his neck. It weighed eight pounds and hurt him so that he carried it on his shoulders in a towel, like a sack. The amputation made by the pair of us was fortunate and the patient recovered.

Cancer of Breast (MI,352)

Being called to open the body of a deceased Great Lady, I found in one of her breasts a tumor the size of a hen's egg, hard and compact as a stone, tough, fibrous and white. While she lived the Physicians and Surgeons considered it a cancer because of its hardness which caused great pain when compressed gently.

---

[14] Dr. Olivier de Violanes from Troyes, received his degree in Medicine in Paris on December 10, 1558 (Le Paulmier).

Breast Tumor (MI,352)

Another time I was called for a similar reason to see an honorable and wise lady where several Physicians and Surgeons had diagnosed cancer and I held otherwise. This tumor was not deeply adherent, there was no unusual color, no enlarged vessels, nor other true signs of cancer. Also, the lady's periods were regular, her complexion and nutrition were well maintained and she had no pain unless pressure was made on the tumor. Moreover, the tumor did not grow nor any other evil develop; on the contrary, she is gay and well disposed, both in body and in spirit.

Retroperitoneal Abscess (MI,356)

Isabeau Rolant, wife of Jehan Bony, living on rue Monceaux near St. Gervais at the sign of the Red Rose, aged 60 years on October 22, 1578, was examined after death by the order and in the presence of M. Milot,[15] Regent Physician and Lecturer to the Schools of Medicine. The pancreas and mesentery were found marvelously and almost unbelievably enlarged, weighing ten and a half pounds. It was hard everywhere and adherent only to the lumbar vertebrae and anteriorly to the peritoneum, which was equally scirrhous, resembling cartilage.

On the following day this was dissected and demonstrated at Dr. Milot's house in the presence of M. de Varades,[16] Physician and Councilor of the King and Dean of the Faculty of Medicine, M. Brouet,[17] King's Physician

---

[15] Beyond this reference by Paré, I could find no other information.

[16] Dr. Jerome de Varades, Physician of Kings François I, Henri II, François II and Charles IX. He was on the staff of Hôtel-Dieu in 1573.

[17] Dr. Gerard Brouet, Physician-in-Ordinary of Kings Charles IX and Henri III.

and Monseigneur the Cardinal de Bourbon;[18] Regent Physicians of the Faculty of Medicine, Messers. Cappel, Marescot,[19] Aragon,[20] Baillou,[21] Riolan,[22] Master Surgeon Pineau,[23] I was also present there, and several others. In it was found a number of abscesses, each having its own cysts some filled with liquid resembling olive oil, others like gruel, others albuminous, and others watery; in brief, there were as many abscesses as types of matter.

But it was notable that the tumor had developed eight or more years earlier, had grown slowly and never was painful. In fact, the mesentery has no feeling. The patient had bowel movements as naturally free as if in full health until two months before she died, when she took to bed because of a fever that continued until her death, also because of the weight of her burden which had the feeling of coming apart. In fact, it was adherent to the lumbar verte-

---

[18] Charles, Cardinal de Bourbon, brother of Antoine, King of Navarre and Louis, Prince de Condé.

[19] Dr. Michael Marescot, born near Lisieaux August 10, 1539, became Rector of the University in 1564, Doctor in 1566, Dean of the Faculty of Medicine in 1588 and Premier Physician of King Henri IV. He was a member of the Commission appointed to examine prior to publication, the second Edition of Paré's *Oeuvres* in 1578 (Le Paulmier, p. 99).

[20] Dr. Euverte de Aragon, Regent Physician, Faculty of Medicine, Paris.

[21] Dr. Guillaume de Baillau, Regent Physician, Faculty of Medicine, Paris.

[22] Dr. Jean Riolan, born at Amiens, became a physician on August 20, 1574 and Dean of the Faculty of Medicine of Paris in 1586. He publicly ridiculed the College of Surgeons for admitting Paré, a Barber-Surgeon, to its ranks and later published a charge of plagiarism against Paré on publication of his "Anatomy." He died on October 18, 1606. A generation later his son, Jean, Jr., a famous anatomist, entered into controversy with William Harvey over the circulation of the blood.

[23] Juan de Pineau, Sworn-Surgeon of Paris, listed in 1547 as the Surgeon of Catherine dé Médicis.

brae alone and to the peritoneum, as described above and not to the bowel or any other part to which it was naturally attached. Lying upon and compressing the bladder, it had caused difficulty of urination and pressure on the bowel had caused difficulty of going to stool, so she needed laxatives. Enemas could not enter; suppositories did no good. She also had difficulty in breathing, because of pressure on the diaphragm. Some of the Doctors considered it a mole, others an hydrops; in fact, hydrops developed; a pail or more of water was drawn from her body. The liver was hard and filled with abscesses, as much within as without. The spleen was decayed, the bowel and omentum livid and speckled; briefly, no part was found healthy in all the lower belly.

Surgery of Cancer of Lip   (MI,365)

Sometimes one may otherwise and more happily cure cancers of the lip without applying caustics or any similar thing after the section and even with little deformity of the part after healing. Such a method I fortunately practiced on a man of fifty in the presence of H. Hautin,[24] Regent Physician in the Faculty of Medicine, a man well versed in medicine, of Jacques Guillemeau,[25] and of M. Eustace,[26]

---

[24] Dr. Jean Haultin, Regent Physician of the Faculty of Medicine, Paris, 1594. He was an intimate friend of Paré, was present when his infant's gums were lanced and assisted at the famous delivery by version of Paré's daughter, Mme. Simon in 1599. According to Guy Patin, he was the real translator of Paré's "Complete Works" into Latin (Doe, p. 157). He died on June 14, 1615.

[25] Jacques Guillemeau was born in Orleans in 1550 into a family of surgeons. He was a favorite student of Paré and lived in his home for a long time. He also served the armies and was Surgeon-in-Ordinary of Kings Henri III, Henri IV and Louis XIII. He was Provost of the

King's Surgeons and of Jean le Jeune, Surgeon of M. de Guise. The way is this: Pass a threaded needle through the cancer so the thread held in the left hand can lift and control the cancer without any of it escaping. One can then cut to good flesh with scissors in the right hand; and cut so that a layer of good flesh of the lip remains to serve as a base and foundation for regeneration of flesh in place of the portion amputated, supposing the cancer has not taken root and spread from top to bottom. This done, having let enough blood flow from within and without, at the right and left of the amputation, make deep enough incisions with the razor so that later, when one would draw together and unite the edges of the wound, as in the case of harelip, the flesh would be more obedient to the thread and needle. The remainder of the treatment is the same as to be used in case of harelip, of which we shall speak later.

Cancer of Breast; Improper Treatment
(MI,370)

I shall give the history of Mme. de Montigny, a Maid of Honor of the Queen-Mother, who had a cancer the size of a nut in the left breast. This caused deep stabbing pains and

---

College of Surgeons on October 1, 1595. He is one of those credited with translating Paré's "Complete Works" (1579) into Latin (1582), but he published it, and attributed the translation to "one who preferred to remain anonymous" (Doe, p. 157). He wrote the best Renaissance book on ophthalmology, *Traite des Maladies de l'oevil*, Paris, 1585, according to Garrison. In 1599, Guillemeau saved the life of Paré's daughter, Anne Simon, suffering a puerperal hemorrhage, by delivering the child by version, as he had learned to do from her father. He died on March 3, 1612.

[26] M. Eustace (other details unknown) witnessed Paré's embalmment of King Charles IX on May 31, 1574.

great pain when pressed upon. One day she spoke of her illness to the Queen, who advised her to place herself in my
hands for treatment. When she showed it to me and told
me how and when the pain was worst, I knew it to be a cancer. I persuaded her to go with me to M. Houllier, Regent
Physician of the Faculty of Medicine, recognized and
known by all as a wise man. When he had examined the
lady he considered the tumor to be cancerous and we decided upon a palliative course, fearing to irritate this Hydra,
and cause it to burst in fury from its lair. He ordered his
regimen and certain purgations which should be used on
alternate days, and on the tumor was placed a sheet of lead
covered with quick-silver. Certain unguents were ordered
for a period of two months. Finally the Lady became rest-
less, since her illness had not been cured nor got worse, and
saw a new Physician. When he saw her tumor, he unwisely
(although he should have known better) promised to cure
her. This made her very happy and she told the Queen of
it. She wanted to know of the Doctor if he found the lesion
incurable; he promptly responded "No" and that he would
cure it quickly. Then the Queen told him, "I am certain
this is an incurable cancer"; nevertheless he persisted and
promised a quick cure.

He rejected our remedies and applied hot applications,
emollients and astringents. The tumor then enlarged
hugely and with great pain and inflammation so the breast
burst like a ripe pomegranate. This was followed by such
profuse hemorrhage that the Doctor, attempting to stanch
it, applied caustic powder which so augmented the pain and
inflammation that the heart failed and death followed. And
so as the Doctor had promised, the treatment was rapid, but
it was the wrong kind.

I wished to recite this history to instruct the young Surgeon so he will not fall into this error.

Axillary Aneurysm   (MI,371)

I saw M. Jean Mallet, a Priest of St. André-des-Arts,[27] who lived at the house of M. de Thou, first President. This Priest had an aneurysm the size of a nut under the shoulder joint and I advised him against having it opened, at the risk of his life. On the contrary he should use *de bolo* ointment and compresses wet with juice of nightshade and honey-suckle mixed with fresh cream cheese and other cold, astringent things. As a protection against rupture, I advised a lead plate and that he wear shorter breeches so his doublet would act as a sling to hold it up. Also that he avoid everything that excites the blood, even that he avoid chanting in full voice at St. André, and he agreed gladly. These things he did for a year, but in spite of it, the tumor enlarged. He went to a Barber who thought his aneurysm another kind of swelling and applied a caustic one evening to make it open. The next morning it opened, spurting a great quantity of blood, which frightened him and he begged the wife of the First President to call me to stop it, telling her that I had well advised him that it should not be opened. Before I could get to him, he was dead.

Wherefore I advise the young Surgeon to avoid opening aneurysms, if they are not very small and in safe places. Open the skin, separate the artery, pass a needle threaded with a strong thread under the artery on each side of the lesion. With these tie off the artery, then cut and treat it as

---

[27] St. André-des-Arts, Paré's parish church, was built about 1212 after completion of the city wall by Philippe-Auguste, on a street of the same name, running parallel to the Seine, a block south of Paré's houses on the rue de l'Hirondelle, at the corner of rue de la Hautefeville. In this church Paré was married twice, baptized nine children and buried most of them. He was buried there himself on December 22, 1590, "at the foot of the nave, near the tower." The church was destroyed in the reconstruction of the area in the 19th century, the present Place St. André-des-Arts marking its site.

a simple wound. Let the threads fall away of themselves; nature will produce flesh to close up the artery.

Aneurysm of Pulmonary Artery[28]   (MI,373)

I saw in the body of a Master Tailor named Belanger who lived on St. Michael's bridge at the Sign of the Cock, an aneurysm of the pulmonary artery, of which he died suddenly while playing hand ball, because the vessel broke. I did the autopsy and found a large amount of blood in the thorax. The body of the artery was dilated to admit a fist and its inner coat was bony. I showed this later at the Medical School to several observers, making an anatomical dissection they greatly admired, and put it in my museum of curiosities.

While Belanger lived all his arteries beat vigorously, his whole body felt hot and he often fell with heart failure. M. Sylvius, King's Lecturer in Medicine forbad him wine, having him drink instead water boiled to make it pure. His food was fresh creamed cheese and the same was applied as a poultice for his pain. At night he ate hulled barley to which he added barley meal and poppy seeds. He was purged occasionally with clysters of cooling things or of cleaned cassia alone. And Belanger told me that of all physicians, he got his greatest help from M. Sylvius.

Hydrocephalus   (MI,377)

I have seen four children ill with this disease of the head, on one of whom I made a section after death. I found the

---

[28] An aneurysm of the pulmonary artery remains an extremely rare lesion. In his critique, Malgaigne was convinced of the authenticity of the observation.

brain no larger than a tennis ball. I have never seen one recover when the fluid is very abundant within the head, but when it is external, recovery is expected.

Empyema (MI,393)

Benedict de Vallée, native of Turin,[29] aged twenty-five years, fell ill of pleurisy which suppurated and made an empyema. He coughed severely, expectorating fetid pus for six weeks; then it ceased for twenty days, at the end of which when he bent over or shook himself, one heard a sound in his body like a half-filled bottle. For the treatment of this he called several Physicians, le Grand, Le Gros, Duret, Liébaut,[30] Violaines and Malmedy, who ordered several treatments. Finally he called me, and having studied his illness, I advised him to have a rib opened to drain the pus. He agreed to do this when he was a little stronger. Some days later nature drained the pus by great vomiting, following which he recovered completely, by the grace of God and of Nature. At present he is as well as if he had never been ill.

---

[29] Turin (Torino), a city in the Italian Piedmont, the scene of Paré's first military experience. Held by the Emperor, Charles V, François I sent an army under the Constable Montmorency to take in it 1536. The mission accomplished, Paré's chief, René de Montejan remained as Governor of Piermont for two years. Here Paré first learned to avoid the use of hot oil in gunshot wounds, the writing of which paved his way to surgical fame.

[30] Jean Liébault, of Langres, was licensed in Paris February 4, 1561. He was a pupil of Duret and married a daughter (Nicole) of Charles Estienne, the printer-Physician, with whom he published several books. Liébault fell into disgrace when his father-in-law was imprisoned for his Huguenot activities (see Le Paulmier 234). He retired to Dijon where he died on June 21, 1596.

Paracentesis for Ascites, fatality from
(MI,400)

I once saw a victim of dropsy who stabbed his belly with an awl to let out the water. He rejoiced to see it flow and his belly deflate. It was impossible to stop the flow and the poor patient died in a few hours because the incision was not made properly.

Hernia Cured with Truss   (MI,407)

There was a Priest of St. André-des-Arts named M. Jean Moret, Epistolier, that is to say, who chanted the Epistle on Sunday, who had a complete intestinal hernia. He came to me, showed me his lesion and demanded help, because when he sang the Epistle especially, he suffered great pain. Seeing his trouble, I told him he really should have another serve in his place. This he did, praying the Curé (M. le Clerk, Dean of the Theological Faculty) and the Church Wardens to employ another, in view of his disability. This they did and he put himself in my hands and I ordered appropriate remedies, having him wear a truss, which he wore for five or six years. One day I asked how he was and he replied that he was cured. That I could never believe, had I not seen it. When I examined him, I found no sign of hernia, a great wonder considering his age, when few are cured. But six months later, advised that he had died of pleurisy, I went to the house of the Curé where M. Moret had lived and begged him to let me open the dead body and learn what obstruction nature had made in the passage through which the intestine had descended. He permitted me to do this. I vow by my God that I found around the peritoneal passage an adipose substance the size of a small tennis ball, infiltrated and attached so firmly that it was difficult to tear it away without tearing and lacerating the adjacent parts. This is the reason the cure resulted.

Undescended Testis Mistaken for Hernia
(MI,418)

At this point I want to advise the young surgeons that sometimes the testes are not yet descended into the scrotum. They are retained in the groin and make a painful tumor, and since it is considered an intestinal hernia, it is treated with astringent plasters, trusses and bandages to restrain it. This increases the pain and prevents descent of the testis.

Not long ago I was called to such a case and after finding a single testis in the scrotum, the child not having been castrated, had the plaster and the truss he wore removed. I told the father to let the child run and jump to help the testis descend into its natural place, which it did little-by-little; without any complication.

Swelling of the Knee   (MI,423)

I remember that M. Greaulme,[31] Regent Physician in the Faculty of Medicine of Paris, had a tumor of the knee composed of mucous and foamy fluid that caused unbearable pain. He had to stay in bed and use many unprofitable remedies. He called me to know if it should be opened. Having examined and felt it, and considering that I found

---

[31] Paré mentioned M. Robert Greaulme and "Greaume" as a consultant, on five separate occasions. He described his death in one case report (see p. 22). Greaulme was mentioned as a Regent Physician in the Faculty of Medicine in Paris, but I can find no other reference to him. Whether or not they all were the same man in conjectural.

no sign of suppuration, I begged him to have more pa-
tience; if it was opened he would regret it, as I had seen
several times. Nevertheless, he had a potential cautery
applied, which greatly increased the pain, with such swelling that the bone got out of place. It was more than two
years before he could stand on his leg and he regretted a
hundred times an hour he had not taken my advice. The
pain diminished a little in time, giving him a stiff leg on
which he limped very painfully. Finally he died of pain and
despair.

Ligature of Bleeding Artery   (MII,8)

A Carter of this city was thrown from his cart falling
headfirst on the pavement. This caused a large contusion
over the posterior part of the parietal bone. When this
was opened to evacuate the blood and to examine the bone,
the incision cut an artery. The surgeon did not know how
to stop the bleeding and the carter lost so much blood he
could hardly turn in bed and scarcely speak, he was so
feeble and debilitated.

I have recited this history to instruct the young Surgeon
that he should not let a man die for fear of the prick of a
needle.

(This history was preceded by a description of a method
of transfixing the scalp layers with a suture to control such
a bleeding artery—ED.)

Compound Frontal Fracture, Cure by Trephine   (MII,16)

One of the servants of M. Gralo (King's Councilor) was
kicked by a mule, the horseshoe fracturing the frontal bone.

Having been called to treat him, knowing the bone to be depressed, I made a triangular incision to apply the trepan. The next day I trepanned to elevate the depressed bone, wishing to extract and remove the fragment; I discovered the great extent of the fracture, which extended from the middle of the forehead to the lesser corner of the eye. Beginning to elevate it so it no longer compressed the dura, discharge flowed from the trepan opening and the dura began to pulsate. I therefore told M. Gralo, who was very interested in the servant's treatment, that despite the severe pain and the extent of the fracture, he could recover. Finally, by God's grace, he recovered, except for loss of the eye on the side of the fracture.

Free Skull Fragment, Replaced (Compound Fracture)   (MII,19)

As Celsus recommended, I treated Captain Hydron of this city who recently was wounded by a sword-stroke in the center of the frontal bone. The bone was cut down to the dura three fingers long and wide so it hung over his face, held only by the pericranium and the muscular layer about three digits wide. Seeing the wound, I decided to remove the bone completely. I recalled then that Hippocrates and other good practitioners had always advised against leaving the brain uncovered if possible. I wiped away the blood covering the cura mater, which I could see pulsating strongly, turned the piece of separated bone and replaced it. To hold it better I sutured the overlying parts in three places and left little packs in the wound to drain the discharges. On this treatment, with the grace of God, he recovered, despite the fact that he had several other serious sword wounds of the thigh, the face and another entering the right side of the chest, going along the ribs and emerging at the side of the tip of the scapula.

Contra-Coup Brain Injury   (MII,21)

It is possible for one side (of the brain—Ed.) to be injured when the other side is struck. This has been observed many times and only recently in one of the servants of Post-Master M. Mats, who was hit by a stone on the right parietal bone with a little cut and great contusion and swelling. This was incised to enlarge the laceration and evacuate the blood in the swelling. This was done by the deceased Thierry de Héry,[32] who never failed to do his duty, since he kept God before his eyes and he was well experienced in surgery.

After the incision was made he saw that the bone was intact. Nevertheless he had a great suspicion that the bone was fractured, since when hit the patient fell unconscious on the ground and vomited, and had other signs indicating fracture. The patient died on the twenty-first day and persuaded by M. Mats, Thierry asked me to seek the cause of death. Opening the skull, we found the bone fissured and

---

[32] Thierry de Héry studied at the Hôtel-Dieu with Paré and followed the French army to Rome as a Barber-Surgeon in 1537, while Paré was in Turin. In Rome de Héry studied syphilis at the Hôpital St. Jacques. Returning to Paris he studied under Jacques Houllier and Antoine Saillard. He and Paré were examined and licensed as Master Barber-Surgeons together in 1542. They dissected together preparing for publication of Paré's book on "Anatomy." In 1544 de Héry was at Jalons with the army. Finally he was named lieutenant of the Premier Barber-Surgeon. Paré described him as a skillful surgeon. He was successful in practice, amassed a considerable fortune and published La Méthode curatoire de la Maladie Vénérienne, Paris, 1552. According to a note by Paré in his L'Anatomie de la tête humaine, de Héry had died before the publication of the book in 1561.

split on the side opposite the blow, a great quantity of bloody pus in the dura mater and even in the substance of the brain; we found no cranial suture except the two squamosals.

Fracture Skull, Inner Table   (MII,22)

A Gentleman of the Company of M. d'Estampes[33] was wounded on the breach of the castle at Hesdin (July, 1553 —Ed.) by a gunshot wound in the parietal bone. A helmet he wore was dented but not pierced by the ball. Neither the scalp nor the external skull was broken, but he died apoplectic on the sixth day.

Wanting to know the cause of death, I opened the skull and found the inner table fractured and splinters of bone driven into the brain although the outer table was intact. I showed a similar case to Drs. Chapelain,[34] Premier Physician of the King and Castellan,[35] Premier Physician of the

---

[33] Estampes, duc d'Jean de Brosse, husband of the Duchesse Anne de Pisseleau, mistress of King François I. He was Governor of Brittany in 1545 when the English attempted a landing at Landerneau. Paré went by post with Mm. de Rohan and de Laval to secure the place. The English withdrew without a fight, but Paré recounted interesting tales of the trip in his "Apologie and Treatise." He was sent home with substantial gifts from the noblemen.

[34] Chapelain, Dr. Jean. Jean Chapelain became a physician of Montpellier and of Paris on April 8, 1541. He was appointed Physician-in-Ordinary by François I and became Premier-Physician of Henri II and Charles IX. Paré so highly esteemed him that he dedicated his book on "Head Injuries" to him in 1561. He died of the plague at the siege of St. Jean d'Angély on December 5, 1569, in the same house where Dr. Castellan, Premier Physician of the Queen-Mother had died of the same disease a month earlier. (Le Paulmier.)

[35] Castellan, Honoré Duchastel (called Castellanus). Physician at Montpellier in 1544, then Professor; was Physician-in-Ordinary of Kings Henri II, François II and Charles IX, then Premier-Physician of

Queen, in a Gentleman who was wounded at the assault of Rouen[36] (1562—Ed.).

King Henri II, Fatal Accident   (MII,25)

All such complications for the most part were seen shortly before the death of the late King Henri II.[37] In a tournament he received a terrible blow on the chest from a tilting lance which opened his visor and the shaft of the lance struck him contra-coup above the right brow, lacerated the forehead transversely to near the inner corner of the left eye, several little fragments or splinters of the lance being embedded in the eye, without facturing any bone. This caused so much commotion and shaking of the brain that he died eleven days after he was struck.

After his death a quantity of blood was found collected

---

the Queen-Mother. Paré dedicated to him his book on the "Plague" in 1568. A year later (November 4, 1569) Castellanus died of the plague at the siege of St. Jean d'Angély. Dr. Chapelain, King's Premier-Physician died in the same house, of the same disease a month later. The next year (February 3, 1570) his son Alexandre became King's Secretary. His sister Louise was the mother of André DuLaurens, who became Premier-Physician of King Henri IV.

[36] Rouen, the city of Jeanne d'Arc's martyrdom in Normandy. In 1562 the Huguenot-Catholic war broke out everywhere. Rouen declared for the Huguenots and was besieged, falling on October 26th. There the King of Navarre (Antoine de Bourbon) received the shoulder wound, of which Paré wrote the interesting account. On his way to Paris from Rouen, Paré was poisoned "for the Religion," but he kept secret the identity of those who attacked him.

[37] Henri II (1519-1559), second son of François I, became King in 1547. Married Catherine de'Médicis, but was more devoted to his mistress, Diane de Poitiers. The intrigues of their partisans promoted the divisions of the Royalty leading to the Religious wars. Father of Kings François II, Charles IX and Henri III. Appointed Paré Surgeon-in-Ordinary at Rheims, August, 1552. Suffered tilting accident June 29, 1559; treated by Vesalius; died July 10, 1559.

between the dura and the pia mater in the area opposite the blow, near the suture of the occipital bone. The substance of the brain was altered and yellow or jaundiced over an area the size of a thumb. Here putrefaction was beginning, which was sufficient cause for the death of the Lord, and not the eye wound. Several have attributed his death to this, but we have seen many who have received worse eye wounds than this and are not dead.

Tilting Wound of Orbit (MII,25)

Similarly recently M. St. Jean, the King's Squire, was in a tournament held before the Hôtel de Guise. He was wounded by a lance splinter the size of a finger under his visor, entering the orbit under the eye penetrating the head about three inches. I treated him under orders of the late King Henri with the good assistance of several Physicians and Surgeons, among whom were M. Valeran, King's Physician-in-Ordinary, Loys Duret and Rodolphe de l'Or, Regent Physician of the Paris Medical Faculty and Jacques le Roy, King's Surgeon-in-Ordinary. Despite the wound made by such a hard blow, he recovered with God's help.

Lance Injury, François de Guise[38] (MII,25)

(Paré has been credited by several writers with the treatment of this wound. Paré never mentioned being

---

[38] Two of the great Guise family were Paré's contemporaries. The first, François, was born at Bar-le-Duc on February 17, 1519, the son of Claude, Comte de Guise, de Lorraine and d'Aumale, and Antoinette de Bourbon. His older sister, Marie, married James V of Scotland and their daughter, Mary Stuart (Queen of Scots) was wife of the short-lived King François II. Charles de Guise, François' brother was second

responsible for the care, and considering his later admiration for the duc, this makes it unlikely. Dr. Regnier, the duc's own Surgeon is the more likely person responsible —Ed.).

In this matter one must not omit the terrible wound received by M. François de Lorraine, duc de Guise (at this time, 1545, he was but comte d'Aumale, not becoming duc until the death of his father on April 12, 1550—Ed.) before Boulogne[39] from the stroke of a lance. This entered under the right eye, declined toward the nose and came out the other side between the ear and the neck, with such violence the head of the lance was broken off with part of the shaft and remained in place. It could be withdrawn only with great force, using blacksmith's tongs. Despite this great violence by the blow of the lance that fractured

---

Cardinal de Lorraine under Henri II and another, Louis, became Cardinal de Guise in 1558. His brother Claude was duc d'Aumale.

At first known merely as Prince de Joinville, François became a famous warrior and general. He received a lance thrust of the face at the siege of Boulogne (p. 167) in 1545 that gave him the nickname "Balafré," or "scar-face." Paré was credited with treating this wound, but he merely described it, never claiming it a personal triumph. On the death of his father in 1550 François became duc. He organized the defense of Metz in 1552, the success of which broke the power of Emperor Charles V, leading to his abdication. In the earlier Religious wars the duc and his brother the Cardinal were towers of Catholic strength. On February 18, 1563 the duc was assassinated by Jean Poltrot, a Huguenot.

[39] With Calais, Boulogne was an important city in the wars between France and England. Paré first went there in August of 1545 when he witnessed the wound of François de Guise made by a lance thrust through his open visor. Although Paré has been credited with this successful case, he never admitted having been other than an onlooker. He apparently visited the camp again in 1550, since on reissue of his book on anatomy printed a year earlier, he apologized for its inaccuracies on the ground that he was at Boulogne when it came from the printer. The city was recovered by France at the peace signed in 1550.

bone, nerves, veins, arteries and other structures being torn and shattered; thanks to God, the duc recovered. (See also pg. 167)

Liver Abscess after Head Injury   (MII,31)

Sometimes an injury to the head causes an abscess of the liver. This Robert Greaume, Regent of the Faculty of Medicine, and Binosque,[40] Sworn Surgeon at Paris and I have seen recently in three patients. If you object that such abscesses were there before the blow was given, I reply that before injury the patients had a healthy and natural color, without any signs of being liverish and were well disposed, doing all their duties. One can learn by experience by taking heed of it, as I did. The cause of this can be that Nature, feeling offended by the great violence of the blow, collects and draws to its aid forces and virtues (which are the blood and the spirits) from all parts of the body toward the heart and liver, as we see in the case of fear and dread, and that causes inflammation of the liver. Thus as happens in some part when the blood flows in greater amount than needed for nourishment, the liver has received more blood and spirits, which can't be utilized because of the scantness and constriction (that is to say for the smallness and narrowness of the vessels), develops fever and phlegmonous swelling it is substance, which causes death. But, if you like better to say with M. de la Corde that Nature succumbs under the burden of illness, undertakes to remove a part of the purulent material with the least effort it can to the liver by the

---

[40] Isnard Rostan de Binosque (Binosc), a surgeon from Provençe who began working with Paré around the time he returned from the siege of Metz in January, 1553. He collaborated in the preparation of the *Anatomie Universelle* of 1561. He died on October 17, 1562.

veins, and by all of which an abscess forms in the liver, the brain-injured patient dies.

(Malgaigne states that this is the first report made of liver abscess following head injuries—ED.)

Massive Blood-Letting in Treating Head Injury   (MII,37)

When discussing bleeding, I do not want to fail to mention this story, worthy of note by all Surgeons. Some time ago I was called to the Fauberg St. Germain-des-Prés, at the sign of St. Michael, to the house of M. Jean Matiau, to visit and treat a young man of about twenty-eight years, of sanguine temperament, servant of M. Douradour, one of the Masters d'hôtel of Madame l'Admiral Brion. He fell on his head on a stone producing in the left parietal area a contused wound without fracture of the bone. Because of this he developed a continuous fever on the seventh day, with great phlegmonous inflammation caused by the lesion of the pericranium, accompanied by an amazing swelling of the whole head and neck, so disfiguring his face that he could not see nor speak. He could swallow nothing but liquids. Upon seeing these complications, although knowing that the day earlier, which was the eight day of his wound, he had been bled by Germain Agace, Master-Barber of St. Germain, of four palettes of blood; seeing such great complications, the patient being vigorous and strong, I drew fourteen more palettes of blood this time. The next day, seeing that the complications and the fever had not abated the slightest and were seen increased, I repeated the bleeding and drew four more palettes, making twenty-two. The next day, seeing that the complications were no less, I again wished to bleed him but did not dare do this alone, considering the volume I had removed. I then asked M. Violaines, Regent Doctor of the Faculty of Medicine, a learned man of good judgment, to see the patient. When he felt the strong robust pulse, and saw the great swelling and the impetuosity and vehemence of the inflammation, he advised prompt bleeding. When I told him I had already drawn twenty-two pallettes, he said, "Even so, if even more had been drawn, it is necessary to draw more. Notice that the two principal indications for drawing blood are present: the seriousness of the illness and the constant strength of the patient." Being pleased with this, I blew three palettes in his presence and would have taken more, but he wanted to wait until after dinner. Then I drew two more, which made twenty-seven palettes taken from the same patient in four days. That night the patient slept well; the next day he was free of fever, the swelling subsided, the inflammation nearly all cleared except in the upper lids, and the ear lobes, which had ulcerated, drained a large quantity of pus. I declare that he was entirely cured, thanks to God, without whose benediction these treatments would have been useless.

(Parés pallettes held about three ounces each, a total of eighty-one ounces, or five pints of blood—Ed.)

Effect of Noise on Head Injury   (MII,38)

I remember when last at the Castle of Hesdin (July, 1553—Ed.), that when they fired the cannon, the noise and vibration of the artillery hurt patients severely, especially those with head wounds. It seemed to them that they were being beaten on the wound with clubs. Sometimes their wounds bled. They made great cries and lamentations and pain, fever and other complications were so aggravated they died quickly.

Large Scalp Avulsions   (MII,39)

If the wound (of the scalp—Ed.) is large enough to require a suture, let as many be used as needed to close it. A soldier in the Hesdin Castle, a little before the last assault (July, 1553—Ed.) was digging earth to take to the ramparts. A large quantity of it fell on him; the soldier was pulled out and his scalp was cut down to the pericranium, the wound starting two inches below the vertex of the skull and the flap hung over his face, making him horrible to see. Having seen him, I called Charles Lambert, Surgeon of the deceased M. le Maréschal duc de Bouillon, to help me treat him.

I washed the wound with wine warmed a little, to remove the blood clot and dirt. Then it was dried with soft linen. I then applied Venice turpentine mixed with a little brandy in which dragon's blood had been dissolved, with aloes and powdered mastic. Then I returned his scalp flap to its proper place and made several stitches, left a little separated to prevent pain and inflammation building up, which happens often when drainage starts. To hold together the parts that were distant and separated, and to prevent entrance of air, which does much harm to such wound, I put long flat tents into the lower edges of the wound so the matter could drain out. Then I applied to the whole head a poultice which is drying, cool and healing, staunching blood flow and diminishing inflammation. He was redressed often, to prevent the farinas in the dressing from drying and closing the pores and thus preventing exhalation and resolution of the vapors contained in the part.

And this soldier was not bled, because he had lost a great deal of blood from the temporal arteries. Being informed that the enemy was ready to attack, I advised him to retire to Abbeville where he could be better treated.

Child Mauled by Lion (MII,41)

But if the wound was made by the bite of a beast, it should be treated otherwise. What I say in this regard is demonstrated by the following history.

One day many were watching the lions kept by the late King Henri[40a] at the Tournelles in this city, one of them escaped and knocked down a girl of about twelve years to the ground with his claws. Then he engulfed her head and made several wounds with his teeth without breaking any bones. She really was being devoured and would have been had not the Master of the Lions saved her from the claws and jaws. Robert Claret, Master Barber-Surgeon of Paris happened to be there and undertook to dress and treat the girl. Some days later I was called to see her. I found her feverish, with great swelling and inflammation of the whole head, shoulder and the chest, chiefly where the lion's teeth and claws had entered. The edges of the wounds were livid

---

[40a] Henri III (1551-1589). This event refers to Henri III, an enthusiastic wild animal fancier.

Edouard-Alexandre, fourth son of Henri II and of Catherine de'-Médicis, became King in 1574 on the death of Charles IX. He was the most detested King in French history, vicious, effeminate and neglectful of his duties. Unable to match the ability and energy of Henri de Guise, he had him murdered on December 23, 1588. The country reacted strongly and he was assassinated on August 1, 1589 at St. Cloud, ending the Valois line. Henri de Navarre succeeded him as Henri IV.

Despite his foibles, Paré served him as faithfully as he had his father and older brothers and retained his post of Premier Chirurgien, Counseiller and Valet-de-Chambre through his reign. Paré survived him by seventeen months.

and they drained serious material, virulent, acrid and so fetid as to be almost intolerable, like carrion, of greenish to black color. The girl suffered severe stabbing and grinding pain. Seeing such complications, I promptly recalled that the ancients had left in their writings that all lacerations and bites of beasts (and those made by men also) were poisoned in greater to lesser degree. So I concluded that it was necessary to let out the poison made by the teeth and claws of the lion and to apply remedies to counteract the poisons. I made several incisions around the wounds and applied leeches to draw out the poison and deplete the inflamed parts. Then I made a lotion of Egyptiacum, methridatum and theriac,[116] with brandy. This was used to wash and poultice all the wounds, and the medication was used in as well as on the wounds, especially the theriac and methridatum. After some time she was for several days given a drink of conserve of roses and Bugloss dissolved in some water and Heart's-ease, to strengthen the heart so it would not become infected by malignant vapors. At the same time a poultice was made to apply over the heart on a scarlet cloth or sponge and removed often. You can be assured that after the first application of these dressings, the pain in the inflammation and the other complications began to diminish and she finally recovered. For more than two years, from being fat and well rounded, she remained thin and slender in all her extremities, but at present she is very well.

Trephine Depressed Fracture of Skull
(MII,63)

M. de la Bretesche, at the entry into Paris of the late King Henri (II—ED.), was wounded by a stone on Nôtre-

Dame bridge.[41] This fractured his petrous bone, with great contusion of the temporal muscle, without a laceration. I was called the next day to treat him in his house at the Red Rose on rue de la Harpe.[42] Having learned the nature of the fracture and the wound, I wished to call consultation with Physicians as well as Surgeons. Some of them advised opening the muscle to apply the trepan to extract the broken bone. I opposed this course on the authority of Hippocrates. In writing on head injuries, he forbade making an incision in such a place, to avoid the accidents mentioned earlier. Also by our own experience, those whose muscle has been cut fall in convulsions and die. But the opening can be made above the muscle, as near the fracture as possible without touching the muscle any more than necessary.

The brother of M. de la Bretesche, one of the Protonotaries of Monseigneur the Rev. Cardinal de Châstillon[43] was present at the consultation for the brotherly love he bore him, and said he would not permit an incision of the muscle, for fear of the accidents described. And thus accord was reached that the incision would be made above the muscle, which I did at once. The next day, which was the third day after injury, I trepanned him and through the opening some days later, drew four splinters of the frac-

---

[41] An ancient Roman bridge across the right branch of the Seine, corresponding to the Petit-Pont on the left. It was burned by the Normans and was rebuilt on piles in 1413. In the 16th century all the Seine bridges were lined on both sides by tall houses affording their inhabitants opportunity to drop objects upon passers-by.

[42] Although an insignificant street now, in Paré's day, rue de la Harpe was a major artery between the Seine and the Porte St. Michel, passing by the Hôtel-de-Cluny and the Church of St. Côme. Much of it has been incorporated into the present Boulevard St. Michel.

[43] Odet, Cardinal de Châstillon (1517-71), nephew of Anne de Montmorency, Constable of France and brother of Gaspard, Admiral de Coligny and of François, Sieur d'Andelot.

ture. I put in a lead pipe or cannula, as the figure shows, to extract the discharge which gathered between the dura and the bone. When dressing him, I had him keep his head low, close his mouth and nose and blow to expell the discharge. Then I washed out the wound with a little syringe shown in the picture and with other remedies; by the grace of God he recovered.

Fungus in Trepan Opening   (MII,63)

A similar case presented itself at the siege of Metz[44] (Dec. 1552—ED.) in the person of M. de Pienne, then called Bugueno. He was injured on the breach (of the city wall—ED.), his temporal bone being fractured by a splinter of stone struck from the wall by an enemy cannon ball. As he was struck he fell to the ground bleeding from nose, mouth and ears, vomiting profusely. For fourteen days he could not speak, respond or recognize anyone. He had frequent tremors approaching convulsions and his face was swollen and livid. He was trepanned at the side of the muscle on the frontal bone by Pierre Aubert,[45] King's

---

[44] Metz was the scene of one of Paré's greatest personal triumphs, of which he wrote a thrilling story in his "Journeys."

In August, 1552, Paré had been appointed Surgeon-in-Ordinary by King Henri II. Foreseeing an attack on Metz, the King sent the duc de Guise there to defend it. The duc worked feverishly to build up the defenses and on October 30th the duc d'Alva besieged the city with 24,000 men. The Emperor, Charles V, arrived on November 20th with 60,000 more. During the desperate fight Paré was smuggled into the city on December 8th with fresh medical supplies and encouragement for the gallant defenders. They did so well that the heart-broken Emperor gave up on Christmas Day and abandoned the siege. Paré shared with the victors the royal honors. The Emperor abdicated his crown on October 23, 1555 in Brussels.

[45] Pierre Aubert, Surgeon-in-Ordinary of Kings Henri II, François II and Charles IX. It is recorded in 1560 that the King gave him 350

Surgeon-in-Ordinary. On the twenty-fifth day a very painful soft mass of flesh called a fungus, grew from the dura mater at the site of the trepanning. This mass increased daily despite the application of corrosive dressings, yet finally he recovered. (See also pg. 170—ED.)

Osteomyelitis of Skull   (MII,66)

At this point I will describe a case I saw when I was in Piedmont[46] as Surgeon of the late Maréschal de Montejan[47] who was then King's Lieutenant. I treated a lackey of the late M. de Goulaines, who was wounded by a sword stroke in the left parietal bone, which did not penetrate the inner table. Some days after his wound was nearly consolidated and healed, a band of soldiers from his country of Gascony arrived in Turin. With them one morning he ate tripe fried with onions and spices and drank a great deal of strong wine

livres tournois in recompense for drugs and equipment stolen from him by soldiers of the late King Henri at the siege of Calais in 1557 (Le Paulmier 191).

[46] Northwestern Italy. In 1536 Paré went there in service of M. de Montejan with the army commanded by the Constable Montmorency, accompanied by the then Dauphin, later Henri II. Turin (Torino) was taken, the Piedmont falling under French control and Montejan was made Governor in 1537. Paré remained there two years, returning to Paris when Montejan died.

[47] René, Seigneur de Montejan (in Anjou), de Sille and de Beaupreau. Colonel-General of Infantry, he took Paré as his Barber-Surgeon on his first army venture in the expedition to the Piedmont of northern Italy in 1536 and was made a Marshal of France the following year. As Paré described in his "Journeys," the Marshal died of liver disease in 1537. Paré so loved him that he refused to serve his successor, the duc d'Annebault and returned to Paris. Montejan's widow, Philippes de Montespedon later married Charles de Bourbon, Prince de la Roche-sur-Yon. She remained Paré's friend and was godmother of his son Ambroise born in May 1576. The child died in January of 1577 and the Princess on October 31st of the same year.

without any water. Soon afterward he developed a continuous fever, lost his speech and understanding; his head and face swelled greatly, his eyes grew red and inflamed and bulged out of his head.

After examining him I called Physicians and Surgeons into consultation to decide what should be done to save his life. With their advice I bled him and gave clysters, applied several medications to his head and massaged and bandaged his extremities. Some days later the area of the wound swelled and when opened drained a large amount of pus. The scalp and pericranium then became depressed, attaching to the edges of the bone which was exposed for about four inches. Finally both tables of the skull became altered, porous, black and rotten. At intervals I applied the cautery to correct this and cause the altered part to separate. About a month after his injury a number of worms came out of holes in the rotten bone. This caused me to hurry the separation of the putrid bone, which had appeared unstable for a long time. On the dura mater, where nature had built up flesh, I found three cavities large enough to admit a thumb, filled with swarming and crawling worms, each about as large as the tip of an aiguilette, and having black heads.

The piece of bone nature had removed was as large as the palm of a hand. To see it one could not understand how nature could cast off so much of the bone of the skull without death, yet finally he recovered, beyond the hopes of all who saw him. After healing of his wound, the scar remained very depressed, as Hippocrates wrote,—and because of this to prevent external injuries, I had made for this lackey a helmet of molded leather which he wore until the scar was very solid and the area reinforced.

Skull Fracture, Loss of Brain Substance
(MII,71)

In the year 1538 when I was in Turin as Surgeon of the late M. de Maréschal de Montejan, I treated one of his pages who was struck on the head by a stone thrown by one of his companions playing quoits. The blow was in the right parietal area, with fracture and separation of the bone so that brain substance the size of half a filbert escaped. Seeing this I pronounced the wound a deadly one. At this, a young Physician came up and argued vigorously against me, saying this was not brain substance but a piece of fat. I told him to keep the stuff while I dressed the patient and I would prove what I had said to be true. After treating the page, to prove by reason and experience that this piece of brain could not be fat, I told him that what is inside the skull cannot be fat although the parts be cold, because of the great quantity of very hot and subtle animal spirits and the heat of the vapors from all parts of the body rising to the head, such things prevent the development of fat. As for experience, in the dissection of dead bodies, fat had never been found there. Yet he wished to gain his end by continuing to protest. Finally I told him that experiments would give us the answer. Several Gentlemen and others present wanted to see this. So I held that if this was fat, it should float in water; contraily, if it was brain substance it would sink. Moreover, if it was fat, it should melt in a hot pan; if it was brain, without frying or liquifying it should desiccate and become dry as parchment and finally burn, because it is stickly, humid and watery. These things were done and proved my assertions. Yet even though the page had lost a part of his brain, he recovered, although he remained deaf thereafter.

Loss of Brain Substance, with Recovery
(MII,71)

Moreover, I have treated two other patients who had lost little bits of brain tisue, with M. Thierry de Héry and the late M. Loys Drouet,[48] experts of great experience in the art of surgery. In these cases mortal signs and complications developed, such as continuous fever, swelling, alienations of mind, scotoma or vertigo, syncope, interruption or irregularity of breathing, redness of the eyes and such. Yet these did not die of their wounds.

Compound Fracture, Brain Extrusion
and Recovery   (MII,72)

Moreover recently M. Étienne de la Rivière,[49] King's Surgeon-in-Ordinary, Loys le Brun,[50] Sworn Surgeon of Paris and I treated M. Robert Courtgenou, one of the

---

[48] Loys Drouet, a Master Barber-Surgeon of Paris, was an early friend of Paré, and witnessed his marriage to his first wife, Jeanne Mazelin on June 30, 1541. He died before the publication of Paré's book on "Wounds made by Fire-Arms" in 1552.

[49] La Rivière was a Barber-Surgeon of Paris. In 1539 he sued Charles Estienne for proper recognition of his part in preparation of an "Anatomy" for publication. The suit was decided in his favor in 1541 and the book appeared in 1545, with him listed as a Surgeon. When a French edition of the book was published a year later, the two were still collaborators. Although Malgaigne termed Estienne "one of the most able Professors of the Faculty," this was a later event; he did not get his degree as a doctor until 1542. La Rivière became Surgeon-in-Ordinary of Kings Henri II and François II and a power in the College of Surgeons, being a member of the Examiners when Paré was admitted in 1554. He and Paré were early friends; he witnessed Ambroise's first marriage to Jeanne Mazelin in 1541; he was the Surgeon to whom Paré went for advice before he substituted the ligature for hot irons to control hemorrhage in amputations, and he was the Surgeon who treated Paré's compound leg fracture in 1561. La Rivière died on July 5, 1569.

[50] Loys, or Louis le Brun, son of Nicholas le Brun, was born in Paris.

Common Chanters of the King's Chapel. He had a sword cut of the frontal bone about five inches long with fracture and complete separation of a piece of bone from the skull. I trepanned him to remove the broken bone which I could not have done otherwise, and after drawing out the piece with special instruments removed others from beneath the cranium. But this bone had torn the dura, and a piece of brain about the size of a filbert or larger, came out in the presence of Messrs. Rosee, Doctor of Theology, Gosselin, Mathemetician and King's Librarian and Claude Rousselet,[51] Bachelor in Medicine. Nevertheless the said de Courtgenou recovered his health and at present is still living.

Blindness from Conjunctivitis, Cured by Seton   (MII,79)

M. Paule, an honest Italian goldsmith living in Nesle[52] near the Augustins in Paris had a discharge from his eyes which several Physicians, Surgeons and others had treated without much help. When he could hardly see to get about he called me and I advised him to go to the extreme remedy, which was the Seton. Having applied it, the ulcer drained sanious material and he began to see better and in measure with the way the ulcer drained, his improvement

He was a licensed Surgeon and with his father, served on the Commission accepting Paré into the College of Surgeons in 1554. He died on November 17, 1581.

[51] Claude Rousselet, Bachelor in Medicine, later Dean of the Faculté, perhaps was a relative of Paré's second wife, Jacqueline Rousselet.

[52] Nesle, a castle and tower at the Seine-end of the city wall of Philippe-August, at present the site of the Institute. A chain stretched from the Tower of Nesle across the Seine to the Tour du Coin of the Louvre to block river traffic. King François I gave Benvenuto Cellini the Little Nesle Castle for a workshop when he brought him to Paris, as he described in his Autobiography. The Convent des Grands Augustins stood east of the tower of Nesle on the present quai of the same name.

continued. After he had carried the Seton for a year or more, he regained his entire vision. Then he tired of it and thinking it of no more benefit, he removed it and let the wound close. But six months later he was in the same trouble, losing his vision as before. Then he called me again, asking me to reset the seton, after which he again regained his vision and has it still at present.

Epilepsy, Cured by Seton   (MII,80)

Recently at the advice of Jacques Houlier, Regent Physician in the Faculty of Medicine, a man of great learning, I applied a seton to a young man of about twenty years of age who often fell with epilepsy. As soon as his ulcer began to drain the falling ceased. It seems true that the virus and the poison is drained by the ulcer made by the seton.

Sword Cut Through Cheek.
Salivary Fistula   (MII,85)

At La Fère[53] in Picardy, two days after the battle of St. Laurence's Day (St. Quentin,[54] 1557—Ed.), I found a

---

[53] La Fère, a small town 24 km. south of St. Quentin. In the 16th century it was an important strong point, but the fortifications are gone. The old Château of Marie de Luxembourg, where Antoine de Bourbon was born is now a rather dilapidated rooming house.

After the battle of St. Quentin in 1557 Paré came here to dress the wounded captured Constable, but the duc de Savoy would not admit him. Paré worked under trying circumstances before returning to Paris. (See his "Journeys in Diverse Places.")

[54] St. Quentin, where on August 10, 1557 the Spanish and English under the duc de Savoy defeated the French. The Constable, Coligny and Montpensier were captured. Condé and de Nevers led the defeated soldiers to La Fère were Paré went to treat them. This victory on St. Laurence's Day inspired Philip II to build El Escorial monastery outside Madrid.

great number of wounded soldiers, among whom was a Gascon who had been cut with a sword across the upper mandible, penetrating the mouth, with great deformity of his face. Because he had not been dressed in the three days since his wound, Binosque, Sworn Surgeon of Paris and I found many worms in the stinking wound. We washed the wound with a decoction of absinthe and aloes with a little Egyptiac, as much to drive out the worms as to remove the discharge. To reduce the swelling of the lips of the wound we applied resolving fomentations and poultices. When resolution was made, Binosque sutured his wound in the manner described above and applied a lotion inside and outside the wound. In a few days the Gascon's wound healed and there remained only a small hole no larger than the head of a pin near the junction of the upper and lower mandibles. From this hole issued a great quantity of clear water when he spoke or ate, as I have often seen before. To stop the flow of clear fluid, we applied aqua fortis to the bottom of the ulcer and sometimes powder of burnt vitriol. By these remedies the wound was healed.

(Malgaigne said this was the first record of a salivary fistula—ED.)

Tongue, Partial Section of Tip   (MII,88)

I was called to the house of the late M. Coüet, Advocate in Parlement, to treat his three year old son who fell striking his chin on a stone. He bit off a good part of the tip of his tongue, which was held only by a bit of flesh. Having little hope that it could unite, I was about to remove it. Considering the very serious effect of inability to speak well and knowing how Nature sometimes does wonderful things, and since the tongue is made of flexible, relaxed and spongy flesh and not subject to injury by air, I changed my mind. I made two sutures, one upward and the other downward and told the mother to nourish the child as described earlier. I assure you that in a few days the baby healed perfectly and at present talks very well.

Suture Tip of Tongue, Recovery   (MII,89)

I can cite a similar recent case of M. Jean Piet, a Carpenter in sound health, living in the Faubourg St. Germain-des-Prés. He fell from a height upon a piece of wood and also bit off the end of his tongue. He came to me to complete the removal, since it hung on very little. In view of the other experience which I have demonstrated, I did not do what he wanted. I sewed it up for him and in a few days he recovered on the same treatment described.

Tracheal Wound, Generalized
Emphysema   (MII,91)

On May 1, 1574, François Brege, a pastry cook of M. de Guise[54a] was wounded at Joinville[55] by a sword cut in the throat. The trachea was partly cut as was one of the jugu-

---

[54a] Henri de Guise (1550-1588), son of duc François. On the assassination of his father on February 18, 1563, Henri became duc de Guise. He assumed his father's role in politics and as champion of the Catholic faith. He even acquired his father's nick-name "Balafré" as the result of a scar left by a pistol shot in the left cheek. He was wounded in the leg at Moncontour in 1569. He finally became so popular that Henri III had him murdered at Blois on December 23, 1588. His brother, Cardinal de Guise was killed the next day.

[55] Joinville, a town on the Marne, of 3500 people, site of a feudal barony. At present the Château-de-Jardin remains, built by duc Claude de Guise, father of François. François was known as M. de Joinville before he became duc. This and Guise were family seats during the 16th century. Here Philip II and the Catholic League signed an alliance against Henri III in 1583.

lar veins, producing profuse hemorrhage and whistling through the trachea. The wound was stitched and astringent dressings applied. Soon afterward the air leaving the wound spread between the muscle spaces and the skin, not of the throat alone but of the whole body, like a sheep inflated for skinning and he could not speak. The face was so swollen that the nose and eyes could not be seen. Seeing these complications all the attendants judged that the said Brege had more need of a Priest than a Surgeon, so Extreme Unction was administered. The next day M. de Guise ordered M. Jean le Jeune, his Surgeon-in-Ordinary to go see Brege, with M. Bugo, celebrated Physician of Madame the Dowager de Guise, as well as Jacques Girardin, Master Barber-Surgeon of Joinville. When they saw him, the Physician could not feel the pulse beating because of the great skin inflation and advised that he be left alone and not to hope for recovery. M. le Jeune, a bold operator having a wide experience and a lively spirit, did not wish to leave the patient without doing something for him. He advised an extreme treatment, to make several deep incisions by which the blood and air were evacuated. Soon the pastry cook regained his speech and sight and after some time recovered completely, by the grace of God. He is still alive, serving M. de Guise in his capacity as pastry cook.

(It is likely that Paré did not participate in the care of this patient, but saw him in October when he went to Nancy to treat Madame Claude de Lorraine—ED.)

Neck Wound, with Brachial Plexus and Vocal Cord Paralysis   (MII,92)

François Prevost, a Nobleman, Ensign of the Coronelle of M. de l'Archan, aged twenty-five years, was wounded by a sword thrust across the throat, passing near the trachea.

It cut branches of the jugular vein and artery from which
ensued great hemorrhage difficult to control. Moreover
one of the speech nerves was cut, as were nerves arising
from the cervical vertebrae going to the arm, so the arm
was powerless and paralyzed. The speech was greatly distorted. The neck remained a little crooked, not letting him
turn as before. Nevertheless he escaped with his life. He
was brought to the house of M. Pierre Pelotot, Master
Barber-Surgeon at the Place Maubert, to be examined and
treated. I was suddenly called there by the patient to dress
him with M. Pelotot. When I arrived and had dressed
him, I had great doubts of his recovery because of the complications he suffered. Because of this I called the experienced Surgeons, Messrs. Cointeret[56] and Piètre,[57] and we
made a legal report of the great hazard against his survival
and that his wound might be fatal. I dressed him to the
end and God healed him. His arm remained powerless and
his speech distorted.

Sword Wound of Trachea and Jugular Vein   (MII,92)

In this regard I want to recite three histories that will be
instructive to young surgeons if such cases fall into their
hands.

---

[56] Jean Cointeret, a Paris surgeon sworn at the Châtelet, died May 13,
1592 (Le Paulmier, pg. 62).

[57] Simon Piètre was born at Varade near Meaux. He received his
degree in 1550 and became Professor and Dean of the Faculté in 1564.
Paré called him an experienced surgeon. He witnessed the autopsy of
Charles IX. He served with Jacquart, Le Comte, Ellain, Rebours and
Marescot on the Commission that approved for publication the Latin
edition of Paré's Oeuvres in 1581. Le Paulmier, pg. 276, designated him
a Huguenot who hid out in the Abbé St. Victoire during the Massacre
of St. Bartholomew. Riolan married his niece Anne.

The first was in 1550. (Malgaigne notes this date an error; Paré had published the case in 1545, but he offered explanations for the confusion—ED.) A servant of M. de Champagne, a Gentleman of Anjou, was wounded by a sword thrust of the throat that cut one of the jugular veins with the trachea. He bled greatly and could not speak until the wound was stitched and treated. But since the medicines were liquid, he drew them between the stitches and passed them through the mouth. Whereof considering the magnitude of the wound and the nature of the wounded parts, principally of the trachea and the jugular vein, which are generative, cold and dry, of themselves difficult to reunite; also that the trachea is subject to movements made in swallowing, because of its external coat being continuous with that of the esophagus, each obedient to the other by a reciprocal motion like a double cord in a pulley; considering also the function of the parts, the trachea serving respiration which is necessary to the symmetry and vital beat of the heart, and that the jugular vein is necessary to the nutrition of the parts above; moreover taking into account the great quantity of blood lost by the wound (which is the Treasure of Nature, conserving the natural heat and vital spirits) and other complications, made my prognosis one of approaching death. Yet I can assure you that he recovered. This I believe due more to the grace of God than by means of the aid of man or of medications.

Throat-cut Patient Talking after Suture of Trachea   (MII,93)

The second history: A while ago two Englishmen lodged together near the Gate of St. Marcel in Paris. One had a sum of money and a large gold chain and some other rich jewels which he ordinarily carried on himself. His

companion wanted to take over these riches and took him
to walk in the forest of Vincennes.. When they were in the
shrubbery he cut his trachea and esophagus and stabbed
him with a dagger. Thinking he had killed him, he left him
stripped to his shirt. Having done this treasonable act, he
hastily returned to the city. Then the victim, who had
feigned death, dragged himself to the house of a peasant
who dressed and treated him and brought him to the city.
One of his companions brought me to treat him. I found
the trachea and the esophagus or gullet (which is the path
of food and drink) entirely severed. I undertook to sew
them up and was able to bring the trachea together end-
to-end, but not the esophagus, which had retracted toward
the stomach. Then I treated the wound with compresses
and bandages. Although he had been speechless, he began
to talk and named his assailant.. The murderer was soon
taken in the Faubourg St. Marcel and finding on him the
possessions of the patient, he was imprisoned and the fact
verified after the death of the patient on the fourth day of
his wound. The murderer was broken on the wheel near
St. Catherine of the Valley of Scholars, the murder being
verified by sewing up the wound of the patient, allowing
him to speak.

Throat-cut, Sutured Permitting Speech
(MII,93)

The third history is similar. A German pensioner of a
banker named Perot, lived in the rue des Noyers in
Paris. In a frenzy one night he cut his throat with a knife
and gave himself other cuts in the thorax and abdomen,
some penetrating through and others superficial. The next
morning some of his companions visited him and found
him very low, with a great quantity of blood around. See-

ing this and believing that his servant who slept in the
room had done it, they sent him to the Châtelet[58] a prisoner
for having murdered his Master. I was called to treat the
wounded man. Seeing the trachea and esophagus cut and
several other wounds, I called Étienne de la Rivière, King's
Surgeon-in-Ordinary and Germain Cheval,[59] Sworn Surgeon of Paris. We decided to suture the tracheal wound as
described above. Promptly after the wound was stitched
and bandaged, the German began to talk and confessed that
he had wounded himself. He absolved his poor servant in
our presence and of several others, including two Notaries
and a Commissioner of the Châtelet. Thus they got the
servant out of prison, entirely cleared by the confession of
the Master. I assure you that solely by surgery was the
German permitted to speak for a period of three days—.

Heart, Stab-Wound; Autopsy   (MII,95)

At Turin I saw a Gentleman who fought with another
who gave him a sword thrust under his left breast penetrating the substance of the heart. He did not cease, but
struck his enemy with many thrusts until he fled. He pursued him a distance of two hundred paces, then fell dead.

On making an autopsy I found a wound in the heart substance large enough to admit a finger, and a large amount
of blood on the diaphragm.

---

[58] Châtelet. An ancient fortress on the right bank of the Seine guarding
the Pont-au-Change. It was mentioned as early as 825 and was enlarged
and strengthened and became the headquarters of the Provost of Paris,
with courts and prisons. It was rebuilt by Louis XIV, but was razed in
1802 and a fountain was installed commemorating Napoleon's victories.

[59] Germain Cheval, an able Surgeon of Paris, was one of the four
Commissioners who examined Paré before his induction into the College
of Surgeons in 1554. He died on May 21, 1570.

Stomach Migrating into Thorax Through Diaphragmatic Wound; Autopsy   (MII,95)

One of these was a mason who was wounded in the middle of the diaphragm in its nervous part, of which he died on the third day. I opened the belly and did not find the stomach. This made me marvel greatly, thinking it a monstrous thing to be without a stomach. Then I considered diligently and realized that it must have entered the thorax even though the wound in the diaphragm was no larger than enough to admit the thumb. On opening the thorax I found the stomach filled with air and containing little fluid.

Colon in Thorax, through Wound in Diaphragm; Autopsy   (MII,95)

A Captain François d'Alon, native of Xantone, was in the troop of M. de Biron, Grand Master of Artillery of France. Before Rochelle he received a gunshot wound, the ball entering at the end of the sternum near the ensiform cartilage, passing through the muscular part of the diaphragm and emerging between the fifth and sixth true ribs on the left side. The wound healed externally but he continued to have a stomach disorder like a sort of colic so he could eat only sparingly. Eight months later he developed a severe colic-like pain in the epigastrium and was treated diligently by M. de Malmedy, Regent Physician of the Faculty of Medicine and King's Lecturer, and M. du Val,[60] Physician of the Faculty of Medicine, men wise in

---

[60] Duval, Dr. Several Duvals were listed among the Paris Physicians at that time. Simon Duval of Rouen, licensed in 1549, Jacques of Evreaux, licensed in 1543 and Antoine, who received his Bachelor's degree in 1567.

Medicine and Surgery. Despite all they could do, he died. I advised an autopsy to find the cause of death and the great pain he had suffered. This was done by Jacques Guillemeau, King's Surgeon, Sworn in Paris, greatly versed in anatomy and other parts of surgery. In the thorax was found a large part of the colon, filled with air; it had entered through a hole only large enough to admit the tip of the little finger, made through the diaphragm by the wound.

Traumatic Broncho-Pleural Fistula
(MII,97)

While in Turin in service of the late M. de Montejan, I was called to treat a Parisian soldier named l'Evesque, under command of Captain Renouart, who was wounded with three severe sword thrusts. One great wound under the right breast penetrated the chest cavity. A great quantity of blood collected on the diaphragm, which impeded respiration and he could speak only with great pain. He had a high fever and with it all he spat blood and had severe pain in his wounded side. The surgeon who first treated him had sewed up his wound so nothing could come out. The next day I was called to see the patient, and seeing the complications and death approaching, I was constrained to open the wound, at the orifice of which I found blood clot. Then I had the patient's legs lifted, with the head and upper part of the body hanging over the bed, resting one hand on a stool lower than the bed. Being so placed I had him close his mouth and nose and inflate the lungs. The diaphragm, intercostal and epigastric muscles contracting, caused the blood collected in the chest to jet through the wound. And to help him do it better, I put my finger deep in the wound to break up the coagulated blood and seven to eight ounces of fetid and corrupt blood drained. Then I put him in bed and injected the wound with barley water in which rose honey and sugar candy had been boiled. Then I had him turned from side to side and finally to lie head down as before. Then one saw little thrombi and clots of blood come out with the irrigation. This done, the complications diminished and little by little, ceased.

The next day I made another cleansing injection, to which was added centaure, absinthe and aloes, but the patient told me he got such a strong bitter taste in his mouth, he wished to vomit. Then I remembered a similar case from the Hôtel-Dieu at Paris, having a fistula of the thorax. Considering that such bitter things soak into the substance of the lungs and through their porosity pass easily to the trachea, to the esophagus and finally to the mouth, is the reason such bitter things should not be used in such wounds, since they bring the patient more unpleasantness than good. But to conclude, this injury was so well handled that beyond my expectation, the patient recovered.

Simple Stab-Wound of Thorax   (MII,98)

Some time ago I was called to treat a German Gentleman at the house of St. Michel on rue St. Denis. He was wounded by a sword thrust penetrating the thorax, which was dressed first by a neighboring barber, who put a large tent into the wound. The next day I visited the German and having seen his wound and examined it to find if blood had collected within, concluded that it had not, since he had no fever nor heaviness and did not spit blood. Then I removed his tent, instilled some of my balm, applied a plaster of diachalciteos and soon he was well. I have done this several times in similar cases.

Wounds of Intestine, with Recovery
(MII,106)

In time I have treated several who recovered after having had wounds by sword or pistol pass through their bodies. One of these, in the town of Melun, was the Steward of the Ambassador of the King of Portugal. He was thrust through with a sword, by which his intestines were wounded so when he was dressed, a great deal of fecal matter drained from the wound, yet the Steward was cured.

Wounds of Intestine, with Recovery
(MII,106)

Recently, I was called to a Parisian Gentleman, M. Gilles le Maistre, Seigneur de Belle-jambe, living in the rue St. André-des-Arts, with Messrs. Botal,[61] Physician-in-Ordinary of the King and Queen and Richard Hubert,[62] Surgeon-in-Ordinary of the said Seigneur, and Jacques Guillemeau, King's Surgeon Sworn in Paris, men learned

---

[61] A native of Asti, in Piedmont, Leonard Botal studied in Paris and Padua, graduating from Paris. In 1564 he was Councillor and Physician of Charles IX, and from 1571 to 1574, of Queen Elizabeth of Austria. He was sent by the King on November 9, 1575 from Paris to Champagne to treat the pistol wound of the face of Henri, duc de Guise, that gave the duc the nickname "Balafré" (scar-face) that had been borne also by his illustrious father, François. The dates of his birth and death are unknown (Le Paulmier).

[62] M. Hubert was described by Paré in various places as a Master Barber-Surgeon, and as Surgeon-in-Ordinary to M. Giles le Maitre, Seigneur de Belle-jambe, and of the King (Charles IX in 1572). Le Paulmier said he died on September 7, 1581.

and experienced in Surgery. The patient had been run through the body by a sword and for several days passed blood by mouth and anus in quantity great enough to indicate the intestines being damaged, yet in fifteen or twenty days he recovered.

Perforating Wounds of the Hand   (MII,112)

As for me, I have treated such wounds differently several times. Of recent memory is that of M. le Coq, Advocate of the Court of the Church, dwelling in the rue Nôtre-Dame, who was at his desk sorting papers, in which was concealed a pen-knife which passed quite through his hand. Also, in case of one of my neighbors, who wished to spit a piece of cold beef, thrust the spit through the middle of his hand. In both I agglutinated their wounds promptly by putting a little of my warmed balm, without a tent, into the wounds at the first dressing. They healed quickly without any complications.

Nerve Injury at Bleeding of King Charles IX   (MII,115)

The King (Charles IX[63]—Ed.) having the fever, M. Chapelain, his Premier Physician and M. Castellan, Phy-

---

[63] Charles IX, third of the six sons of Henri II and Catherine de' Médicis, succeeded his brother François II as King at the age of 10 in 1560, under the regency of the Queen-Mother. A weak youth during the exacting times of the Religious Wars, his was one of the most unhappy reigns in French history. Persuaded by the Catholics, he sanctioned the St. Bartholomew's Day massacre of the Huguenots on August 24, 1572. He was fond of Paré and elevated him to the rank of Premier-Surgeon and Councillor on January 1, 1562. He kept him in the Louvre for his protection on St. Bartholomew's Day. Suffering terrible remorse over his deed, he died of tuberculosis on May 30, 1574 in the thirteenth year of his reign. Paré performed his autopsy and embalmed his body.

sician of the Queen and Premier of the Queen, his Mother, ordered him bled, and to do it, they called one (Portail[64] —Ed.) who had the reputation of bleeding well, who thinking he was opening the vein, pricked the nerve. The King promptly cried out that he felt a severe pain. I immediately ordered the bandage loosened; otherwise the arm might swell quickly. This happened immediately, with a contracture of the arm so that it could not be flexed nor extended freely, and the pain was extreme at the point of puncture as well as through the whole arm. For the first and most prompt remedy, I applied a little plaster of basilicon for fear the wound would clot and over the whole arm I applied compresses wet in oxycrate, with a compressive bandage beginning at the wrist and ending at the shoulder, to drive the blood and spirits to the center of the body, for fear that the muscles would develop too great swelling, inflammation and other complications. That done, we retired to consult and decide what medications we should apply to sedate the pain and to avoid complications which ordinarily follow puncture of nerves. I advised that we should put into the puncture warm oil of turpentine with a little rectified brandy and over the whole arm a plaster of diachalciteos dissolved in vinegar and rose oil, and continue the ex-

[64] Antoine Portail was born in Béarn around 1530 and came in the suite of Jeanne d'Albret to Paris where he studied and became a Master-Barber-Surgeon. He served in the siege of Doullens (1558) when he worked with Paré. Thereafter he married Jacqueline de Prime, cousin of Paré's wife Jeanne. This was the beginning of an intimate relationship that unfortunately dissolved later (Malg. II, 329). Portail was later made a Master Surgeon and Surgeon-in-Ordinary to Kings Henri II, Charles IX, Henri III and Henri IV. Although he injured a nerve in the arm of Charles IX while bleeding him, he did not lose royal favor and was kept at his post by Henri III. He and Pigray[9] were present when Henri III was assassinated on May 13, 1588. The Béarnese King Henri IV made him his Premier-Surgeon and later elevated him to the nobility as Ecuyer. François Martel succeeded him as Premier Surgeon.

pulsive bandage. My reasons were that the oil and brandy could penetrate to the depths of the puncture, dry the moisture from the nerve and by their actual and potential warmth, calm the pain. The diachalciteos plaster had equal virture of resolving the humor coursing the arm and prohibit the descent of other humors. As for the bandage, it served to strengthen and sustain the muscles, express and remove to the upper parts the humors that descend and prevent their new flow. The Physicians agreed to this and concluded such remedies to be useful and necessary. Thus the pain ceased. And to better resolve and slow the humors contained in the part, we used resolving and drying remedies.

The King remained three months and more without power to flex or extend the arm, nevertheless, thanks to God, he was perfectly healed without being deprived of any motion.

Gangrene of Arm after Bleeding Accident   (MII,116)

Of recent memory was Mademoiselle Courtin, living in rue St. Croix, near the Bretonnerie in Paris, who being badly bled, the arm fell into gangrene and total mortification, of which she died, since she was not so treated.

First Experience with Gunshot Wounds   (MII,127)

(1536, Paré's first military expedition under M. de Montejan to Piedmont and Turin, with the army commanded by the Connestable Montmorency and accompanied by the Dauphin, later Henri II.—Ed.)

I was at that time a fresh-water surgeon, since I had not yet seen treated wounds made by firearms. It is true I had read in Jean de Vigo,[65] first book of *Wounds in General,* Chapter 8 that wounds made by firearms are poisoned because of the powder. For their cure he advised their cauterization with oil of elders mixed with a little theriac. To not fail, this oil must be applied boiling, even though this would cause the wounded extreme pain. I wished to know first how to apply it, how the other Surgeons did their first dressings, which was to apply the oil as boiling as possible with the tents and setons. So I took heart to do as they did. Finally my oil was exhausted and I was forced to apply instead a digestive made of egg yolk, rose oil and turpentine. That night I could not sleep easily, thinking that by failure of cauterizing, I would find the wounded in whom I had failed to put the oil, dead of poisoning. This made me get up early in the morning to visit them. There, beyond my hope, I found those on whom I had used the digestive medication feeling little pain in their wounds, without inflammation and swelling, having rested well through the night. The others on whom I had used the oil I found feverish, with great pain, swelling and inflammation around their wounds. Then I resolved never again to so cruelly burn the poor wounded by gunshot. (See also pg. 162—Ed.)

---

[65] Giovanne da Vigo was born in Rapello in 1460. When Julian II became Pope in 1503 he brought da Vigo as his Surgeon to Rome, where he developed a large practice. Following the Pope to the Wars, he worked for ten years on a series of books on Medicine and Surgery. It was published in Rome in 1514 in nine volumes, *Practica Copiosa in arte Chirurgica* and went through 21 (Malgaigne) or 40 (Castiglione) editions including translations into several foreign languages. Malgaigne listed its contents and noted that he originated no single new idea, method or process; it was the work of a compiler and copyist. The man himself passed from sight and his place and time of death is unknown; 1525 is the approximate date (Malgaigne, Intro. CLXXV).

Onion Treatment of M. de Montejan's Burned Scullion   (MII,128)

One of M. le Maréschal de Montejan's kitchen boys fell into a caldron of nearly boiling oil, for the treatment of which I was called. I promptly went to the Apothecary to get cooling medications customarily applied to such burns. A village woman there heard me speak of the burns and advised me, for fear he would not survive the pustules or blisters, to use as a first dressing fresh onions crushed with a little salt. I asked if she had had experience with the dressing and she assured me in her jargon, that she had. This decided me to try the method on the little kitchen boy and truly, I found that the places covered by the onions had no blisters or vesicles, while the other places were completely blistered.

Onion Treatment of Powder Burns   (MII,128)

Some days later a German of M. de Montejan's guard was badly burned. The fire took in his powder-flask so it made a great disaster to his hands and face and I was called to treat him. I applied the onions to half his face and the usual remedies to the other. At the second dressing I found the side where I put the onions without any blisters or excoriations. The other was all burned; then I proposed to write the effect of the said onions.

Pistol Wound Through Thighs, Earl of Gordon   (MII,129)

Not long ago I had an experience with the Scottish Gentleman, Earl of Gordon, Lord of Achindon, whom I treated at the command of the Queen-Mother. He was wounded through both thighs, without fracture of bone, by a pistol shot which was so near him that the fire burned his breeches. He was entirely cured in thirty-two days without having fever or any other complication. I treated him at St. Jean de Latran at the house of the Scottish Ambassador, Archbishop of Glasgow, who daily helped him and watched his treatment. Those who can testify to the truth of this are M. Brigard, Regent Physician of the Faculty of Medicine, who treated him with me, together with Jacques Guillemeau, King's Surgeon Sworn in Paris. The same can be witnessed by M. Hautin, Regent Physician in the Faculty of Medicine, who saw him on alternate days and Giles Buzet, Scotch Surgeon. All marvelled that he healed so well without application of strong or acrid medications.

Bullet Carrying Cloth into Wound
(MII,136)

To prove my statement (that bullets are not hot when they strike—ED.) I will be content with the example of a soldier from whose thigh I remember having removed a ball. It was wrapped in the taffeta of his breeches, producing a deep wound. When I drew it out with the taffeta there was no sign of any burn.

Finding a Buried Bullet: Wound M. de Brissac
(MII,146)

Sometimes it happens that the sound cannot find the ball, as happened at the camp of Perpignan[66] (Aug. 1542—ED.)

---

[66] Perpignan. A city of 70,000 on the river Tet, ten miles off the Mediterranean coast and just north of the Spanish border. In a fight to drive the Spanish and English coalition out of France, François I

to M. le Maréschal de Brissac[67] wounded by an harquebus
shot near the right scapula. Several Surgeons could not find
the ball and thought it had entered the trunk, since it made
no wound of exit. Then I was brought by M. de Rohan to
M. de Brissac to see if I could find the ball. I began to seek
the ball, and not wishing to use the sound again, I asked
him to put his body in the position it was when he was
wounded. Then I gently felt the parts around the wound.
This let me feel a hard mass in the muscle, with a feeling
of pain and fluid where the ball was. It was between the
inferior part of the scapula and the seventh or eighth
vertebra of the back. At this spot an incision was made to
remove the ball, after which he recovered completely. (See
also pg. 165—Ed.)

Pistol-Shot of Elbow   (MII,168)

It should help the young Surgeon to recount this history
of the wound of M. le Comte de Mansfeld,[68] Governor of

---

besieged Perpignan from August 24th to September 4th, 1542. Ambroise
was called into service suddenly and rode horseback by post, so hard that
he suffered an attack of hematuria at Lyon. Apparently he recovered
satisfactorily since he continued his journey and described the lifting of
the siege when the French camp ground was flooded by the rising river.

[67] Charles de Cosse, Count de Brissac, called "The Beau Brissac," was
successively named Colonel of Infantry, Colonel-General of Light
Cavalry, Grand-Master of Artillery, Marshall of France, then Governor
of Picardy. He died of gout December 31, 1563, at the age of fifty-seven
years (Le Paulmier). One of his daughters married the Count de Mansfeld, who fought at Moncontour.

[68] Pierre-Ernest, Count de Mansfeld, married the sister of François,
father of Christopher Bassompierre, who also received a similar wound
in the same battle. Mansfeld was Governor of Luxembourg and a
Chevalier of the Order of the King of Spain, by whom he was sent to
the assistance of Charles IX, to be wounded at Moncontour in 1569.
Being a representative of the Spanish King, Catherine de' Médicis

the Duchy of Luxembourg, Chevalier of the Order of the King of Spain. He was wounded at the battle of Moncontour[69] (Oct. 3, 1569—Ed.) by a pistol shot at the joint of the left arm, fracturing the bone, which was as badly comminuted as if it had been broken on an anvil, because the shot was made at close range. By the violence and force of the blow, several complications developed: violent pain, inflammation, fever, edematous swelling, crepitation of the entire arm down to the fingertips and the great danger of gangrene. To counteract this and complete mortification, several deep incisions were made by M. Nichole Lambert[70] and M. Robert Hubert, King's Surgeons-in-Ordinary.

But by the command of the King (Charles IX—Ed.) I was sent to dress him and having arrived, seeing these complications accompanied by a great stench and corruption, advised that they make irrigations with fortified Egyptiac dissolved in vinegar and brandy, and other remedies written in the Chapter on Gangrene. In addition to these complications, the said Lord had diarrhea, by which he threw off pus which came from ulcers of his arm. Several could not be-

---

insisted that the reluctant Charles send Paré to dress him. Le Paulmier (p. 93) also mentioned Charles de Mansfeld, son of Pierre-Ernest, born 1543, as a godfather of Paré's son Ambroise on May 30, 1576. The godmother was Philippes de Montespedon, widow of Paré's first military chief, the Mareschal de Montejan, but now Princess de la Roche-sur-Yon.

[69] In September, 1569, the Admiral Coligny was forced to raise the siege of Portiers. On October 3rd, he was forced into battle by the Catholic forces under the duc d' Anjou (later King Henri III), on the banks of the Vienne, below Tours. The Admiral was wounded and the Huguenots lost 5-6000 men and most of their baggage. The wounded Catholic noblemen retired to Tours for treatment and Charles IX sent Paré there to treat them.

[70] Surgeon-in-Ordinary of Kings François II and Charles IX, Nicole Lambert was among the witnesses of Paré's autopsy and embalmment of Charles IX on May 31, 1574. He had been a godfather of Paré's short-lived son Isaac, baptized at St. André-des-Arts, August 11, 1559.

lieve this, requiring, they said, that to descent by the bowel, the pus would need be mixed with the blood, which going near the heart and through the liver would cause many complications, which would cause his death. Moreover, it seems to me that I have amply demonstrated in my writing on *The Suppression of Urine,* how such things happen. So anyone who wishes to know the reason can have recourse to that text.

Often the Seigneur swooned from the putrid vapors which arose from the ulcers; which vapors were conveyed by the arteries, veins and nerves to the stomach and the noble parts. To remedy this, I gave him spoonsful of brandy in which a little theriac was dissolved. M. Bellanger,[71] King's Physician-in-Ordinary and M. le Bon, Physician of M. le Cardinal de Guise, wise and expert in Medicine and Surgery, helped at the same time in every way in their power to combat the fever and other complications. To control the edematous and gassy swelling that occupied the whole arm, I applied compresses soaked in oxycrate, with salt and a little brandy and other remedies I thought proper. Then I sewed on doubled bandages as snugly and smoothly as I could, that is to say, as much as the Lord could endure. Such compression served to hold the broken bones in place and to expel the discharge of the ulcers and drive the humors toward the center of the body. When we desisted in binding and supporting the arm, the swelling increased so greatly I was afraid the natural heat of the arm would be suffocated and extinguished. And it was impossible to make any other kind of bandage, because of the extreme pain he suffered when the arm was moved in any way. He developed several other abcesses around the

---

[71] Simon Bellanger was physician of Kings François II, Charles IX and Henri III.

elbow joint and several other places on the arm. To drain the pus I made several incisions which the Lord endured willingly, telling me that if two were not enough I should make three or even four, for the wish he had to be out of his pain and cured. Then smiling I told him that he was worth hurting and not these dainty ones who always prefer to die than to suffer incisions necessary for their recovery. To speed the cure I irrigated the ulcers with a healing solution of Egyptiac dissolved in wine or with rose honey in place of the Egyptiac, to cleanse and correct the drainage, with other remedies too many to mention: among others, powdered alum to dry up the spongy, lax and soft flesh. Also after the ulcers changed, at each dressing I put a dry compress in each hardly smaller than a fist. And one day seeing that he was without pain and that the muscle had healed, I told him he would get well. Then he told me laughing, that he knew it, since now he used compresses no bigger than an egg.

During this cure, I attest having removed more than sixty pieces of bone, some as large as a finger, broken into strange shapes. Notwithstanding this, thanks to God, the Lord was cured, but he could never flex nor extend the arm. (See also pg. 184—ED.)

Pistol Shot of Elbow M. de Bassompierre (MII,170)

M. de Bassompierre,[72] Colonel of twelve hundred horse, the day of the same battle (Montcontour Oct. 3, 1569—

---

[72] Colonel of 1200 Cavalry, M. Bassompierre was shot in the right elbow at Jarnac, crippling the joint. At Moncontour he suffered a similar wound of the left elbow, crippling it also. His son François became a Marshal of France and wrote the *Mémoires de Bassompierre* (Le Paulmier).

Ed.), was wounded by a similar injury and had a great deal the same complications. I dressed him also to recovery, thanks to God. It is true that he had the same disability as the other Lord.

Compound Fracture of Thigh, M. de Croy   (MII,170)

After having treated Messrs. le Comte de Mansfeld and Bassompierre, I was commanded by the King to go quickly and find Charles Philippes de Croy[73] Marquis d'Aurey, brother of M. le duc d'Ascot,[74] near Mons[75] in Heinaut.[76] He had been bedridden seven months or more by a harquebus shot three inches above the knee. I found him with the following complications: intolerable pain, continuous fever, cold sweats, great emotional upset, decubitus ulcer as large as the palm of a hand (from having lain too long on his back), not able to rest night or day, without

---

[73] Charles Philippe de Croy, brother of duc d' Ascot (q.v.), posthumous son of Philippe II, duc d' Ascot and de Croy and of Anne de Lorraine, his second wife, born September 1, 1549. Charles married Dianne, widow of Rhingrave de Dauhn, killed at Moncontour. He was also Marquis d'Havre and was twenty years old when Paré treated him. He died November 23, 1613 (Le Paulmier).

[74] Philippe III, duc d' Arschot, prince de Chimay, born July 10, 1526, son of Philippe II, duc d' Arschot and of Anne de Croy. He was brother of the Marquis d'Auret of Havre (q.v.), Knight of the Golden Fleece and Grandee of Spain. He died on December 11, 1595 (Le Paulmier).

[75] The famous Flemish battlefield of centuries, just above the French border. In the 16th century this area was known as Heinalt or Heinault. In the autumn of 1569 Paré was sent to the Château d' Auret, near Mons to treat the wounded Marquis d' Auret. After completing this successfully, the local people were so overjoyed they took Paré in a triumphal tour of the area, as far north as Antwerp, as he described so delightfully in his "Journeys."

[76] Heinault—an ancient province including parts of northern France, Flanders and southern Belgium.

appetite for eating, but drinking enough. He often sank
into his bed with epileptic fits, was nauseated frequently,
trembled constantly and could not carry his hand to his
mouth without help. He fell often into syncope from failure of his heart, due to the putrid vapors that were conveyed to the stomach and other noble parts by the arteries,
veins and nerves, which were carried from his ulcers and
the decaying bone. For the bone of the thigh was fractured
and split lengthwise and across, with splinters, some of
which had separated, others not. He had a sunken ulcer of
the groin extending to the middle of the thigh, from which
extended other sinuses and canals around the kneecap. All
the muscles of thigh and of leg were extremely swollen
and imbued with a mucoid humor, cold, wet and gassy, so
the natural heat was almost suffocated and extinguished.

Seeing all these complications, his powers prostrate and
greatly depressed, I strongly regretted having been sent
to this Lord, for he gave little sign that he could recover
and I feared he would die in my hands. Still, considering
his youth, there was still some hope, for God and nature
sometimes do things that to the Surgeon appear impossible.
I asked the Lord to have good courage and told him that if
he would endure to have some incisions, which for his treatment were more than necessary, most of his pains and other
complications would clear up. Then he told me he would
endure anything and to amputate the leg if necessary. At
this I was happy, and I made two openings to let out the
matter which was around the bone and in the substance of
the muscles, and which drained a large amount. Afterwards
this was syringed with wine and a little brandy containing
a good quantity of Egyptiac, to clear up the putrefaction
and to dry up the proud flesh, and to resolve and consume
the edematous swelling and crepitation, sedate the pain

and rekindle and strengthen the natural heat which was almost extinguished, because the parts could not assimiliate the necessary nutrition due to the very great amount of pus.

His Surgeon, M. Antoine Mancler of Mons, a man of good and wide experience in Surgery and I made fomentations of sage, rosemary, thyme, lavender, camomile flowers, melilot, and red roses boiled in white wine, with lye made of oak wood, some vinegar and a pinch of salt. This decoction thus made had the virtue and ability of extracting, draining, resolving and drying the cold and phlegmy humor and restoring the wounded parts. These fometations were long continued so the resolution was greater, for being thus made long, resolved more than it could draw, liquified the deep humors, and clearing the skin, as well as the flesh of the muscles.

And with this purpose we made friction with warmed kerchiefs, in all ways, from below upward and from above downward, to right, to left, around and long continued, for brief friction draws more than can be absorbed. On alternate days we put around the thigh, leg and sole heated bricks sprinkled with vinegar and white wine with some brandy. By the evaporation of these, we saw perspiration start from the skin pores, the swelling diminished and the natural heat was restored. Afterward they applied compresses treated with oak-wood lye in which had been boiled sage, rosemary, lavender, salt, brandy and cloves, applied with bandages so dextrously that the patient could well endure them. These were so helpful that when they were omitted for a day the swelling increased. Also large compresses were introduced to the bottoms of the ulcer sinuses to express and displace the pus. And to make them better the orifices of the ulcers were held open with cannulated tents. To help resolve the swelling a specially prepared poultice was applied. At the same time we applied de Vigo's plasters with-

out mercury, which helped greatly to soothe pain and to
reduce swelling. These were applied after the parts had
been warmed by frictions, fomentations and evaporations,
for otherwise the plasters would have been less effective because of the intemperate cold of the parts. But for the modi-
fication of the ulcers we applied proper remedies and
changed them as we saw the need. Also, catagmatic powders
were not spared to make the bone separate and correct its
rottenness. We also used a vulnerary potion for fifteen days.
Every day he had a generalized massage to the whole body,
which was very worn and thin, due to the pain and other
complications that have been described, and also from lack
of exercise. These massages renewed and livened the blood
and resolved some fuliginous humors between the skin and
the flesh. Consequently the parts were thus better nourished,
suppled and refreshed. After the pains and the fevers
passed, he began to sleep well and to have a better appetite,
so we gave him good food and good wine and beer to drink.
He and I shared a hot soup every morning and he became
plump, strong and well, except that he could not bend the
knee very well. (See also pg. 186—Ed.)

I have wanted to give these histories to guide the young
Surgeon in practice, not to praise and glorify myself, but to
render it to God, knowing that all good things come from
Him as from a never-failing fountain and not from our-
selves. By thus giving Him thanks for all good works, I
pray Him to continue and to increase in us His Infinite
Favor.

Astringents in Fresh Wounds   (MII,179)

In this regard I recall having treated a Moor belonging
to M. le Comte de Roissy, who was wounded before

Bologne (1545—ED.) by an Englishman who thrust a lance through his arm. To help stop the hemorrhage, I put in the wound an astringent containing sharp vinegar, for want of anything else. But later he looked me up, saying his arm felt on fire. I was constrained to dress him again and changed the remedy in his wound, applying the astringent outside.

Bleeding From Orifices after Body Wound (MII,195)

Equally for a shot through the body, the blood can leave the vessels, a part of which passes by stool and urine, which I witnessed in the case of the late M. de Martiques. At the last siege of Hesdin (1553—ED.) he wanted to see over the rampart enemies who sapped the foot of the wall. He was struck by a harquebus shot through the body, after which he passed blood by mouth, by anus and urethra, which caused his death. (See also pg. 9 and 171—ED.)

Onions for Skin Burns (MII,204)

I have seen by experience that onions do wonderful things. In Piedmont I treated several soldiers burned by a train of cannon powder made by the enemy at the assault of the Castle of Villaine.[77] I assure you that where I put the onion paste in the manner described, no pustules or vesicles developed as happened to others to whom the remedy was not applied.

---

[77] A castle lying between the Pass de Suze on Mt. Cenis, and Turin. It was held by Imperial troops and was captured by the French army on Paré's first military expedition. He recounted his experiences there in the "Apologie."

Deep Burn of Leg   (MII,209)

That which I have sometimes seen happened recently to a child aged about ten years who was found in a wood all frozen, unable to move or speak, having only a little respiration. After being brought out of the wood he was put near a fire where he was so warmed up that the larger part of one of his legs was burned nearly to the bone. Several, seeing the leg so badly burned, thought the scar would be so large and so hard that it would make the part insensible, and concluded it would be more expedient to remove it. For this I was called, but I promptly scarified it with several deep incisions to which I applied unsalted butter, with rose oil and egg yolks in good quantity to make the crusts come off. Under the knee I put unguentum contritrum, with compresses and bandages treated with oxycrate. These were renewed often to inhibit and prevent the flow of humors which cause pain. After the crusts fell off, I applied album rhasig ointment and poplar salve equal parts, mixed and beaten in a lead mortar. Egg whites were used to stop pain, which stopped. I increased the drying remedies, etc., until the ulcer was full and ready to scar over. Then I bathed the ulcer several times with chalk lotion, using a drying powder after the bathing. As a result, the child was perfectly healed.

Skull Defect with Brain Protrusion
Resembling Aneurysm   (MII,212)

The following history I think remarkable and worthy of great admiration. M. du Fresnay, a Collector for Madame la Connestable,[78] lived in the town of Senlis.[79] He sent for

---

[78] Madame le Connestable, wife of Anne de Montmorency, Connestable of France.

[79] An ancient cathedral town 44 Km. north of Paris, occupied since

me to come see him since he had on his head a tumor the size of an egg between the occipital and parietal bones. He wanted me to open it, thinking it an abscess. I found two Physicians and two Surgeons living in Senlis, honorable and wise men. We consulted on the question of opening it.

Having observed the tumor, realizing that it had developed little by little and was of long standing, and after having felt and noticed a pulsation (which was the movement of the brain) like that of an artery, and when I pressed my hand upon it the tumor abated and diminished, truly I thought this was an aneurysm. Consequently I said that one should be very careful about opening this tumor, for fear of hemorrhage and of sudden death. But one of the Physicians and one of the Surgeons felt there was no danger in opening it, estimating that it only contained pus. The opinion being thus divided, I suggested that we ask the opinion of M. Fabry,[80] Physician-in-Ordinary of the King and of Madame la Connestable, who was then at Chantilly,[81] as to whether it should be opened or not. He promptly gave his advice, estimating as did the others, that it contained only pus and that it could be emptied without danger. Then when I told him that I had the opinion that this was an aneurysm, by the signs I mentioned, he changed his mind and concluded that it should not be touched. The

Roman days. It was here in 987 that the Archbishop of Rheims proposed to the "ducs of France" that they choose Hugh Capet as their King.

[80] Physician of King Henri II and of his children, of Kings François II and Charles IX (after Simon Burgensis, in October 1567) and of Henri III until 1584 (Le Paulmier).

[81] Chantilly—a town 40 Km. from Paris, the site of five châteaus built over 2000 years in the valley of the Nonette. It was the family seat of the Montmorencys. The Château was refurbished in the Renaissance style by the Constable in 1528. After his death it went through the hands of the Condés and is now a state museum.

resolution made, I returned to Paris, but three days later the Collector sent for a Barber of a village near Senlis, who as soon as he arrived and had seen the patient, said the tumor contained pus and that there was no danger in opening it. This he did, and instead of pus, brain substance escaped. Two days later the Collector died. After his death, the head was opened by Adam Hannequin and Hamard Cheron, Master Barbers and Surgeons of Senlis. They told me the tumor consisted of brain substance, with loss of the two tables of the skull as large as the palm of a hand (Noble à la rose).

Sudden Gangrene of Legs (Aortic Occlusion?) (MII,214)

I remember having seen in Paris a man who was feeling well in the evening, not bothered by any pain. During the night he developed gangrene and mortification of the two legs without swelling or inflammation. But in certain spots the color tended to lividity, blackness and greenness, while in some spots the color was almost natural. Moreover they had no feeling and when they were pricked with a lancet or the point of a pin, no blood appeared. There was no warmth to the touch, but on the contrary one felt coldness. Seeing this I called for advice, by which it was decided and ordered that several deep incisions should be made to attempt a cure. This was done, but from the incisions came only a little dark blood, thick and partly congealed. Several other remedies were applied, but nevertheless the patient soon rendered his spirit to God with great suffering, his face and all his body livid. I leave the question if the cause was not poisoning.

Loss of Parts from Cold   (MII,214)

I well remember having treated in Piedmont many soldiers who crossed the mountains in winter. From the extreme cold, some of them had lost ears, others parts of an arm, others their virile members, others toes. Others lost their lives; witness the "Chapelle des Transis,"[82] situated on Mont Senis.[83]

Frozen Leg, Gangrene, Amputation and Death   (MII,214)

In winter a poor Breton stable servant in Paris, after having drunk well, went to bed near a half-opened window through which cold entered. This affected one of his legs so that when he tried to get up, it could not support him. He was put near the fire and thinking his foot merely asleep, he burned the sole nearly an inch deep without feeling anything, for more than half his leg was mortified by the cold. The next day the Breton was taken to the Hôtel-Dieu[84] where he was visited by the Surgeon and others, who

[82] Chapel "of the Frozen," on the pass of Mt. Cenis, in the Alps between France and Italy, dedicated to travellers frozen on the journey in the mountains.

[83] A high mountain south of Mont Blanc in the French Alps between France and the Italian Piedmont. On Paré's first military expedition, he went over the pass here with the army under the Constable Montmorency, in the employment of M. de Montejan and saw his first of soldiers wounded in battle. He suffered a revulsion of war from which he never recovered and to the end of his life dedicated himself to improving the lot of the ignorant and quite helpless common soldier.

[84] Established by St. Landry, Bishop of Paris in the 7th Century, this was the first charity hospital in France. Paré served as a resident Barber-Surgeon for two or three years around 1535, no exact dates being on record. At that time it stood in front of the Cathedral on the river bank between the present Petit-Pont and the Pont-au-Double on the plot now

found it necessary to amputate his dead leg. This was done, but the mortification had reached the upper parts, so in three days the Breton died with cold sweats, ravings, belching and fainting.

Frozen Noses of Patients at Hôtel-Dieu   (MII,215)

That same winter was so very cold that several patients in the Hôtel-Dieu had the tips of their noses mortify without any putrefaction. In four of these I amputated the involved parts, of whom two recovered; the others died.

Re-amputation of Painful Leg Stump   (MII,221)

On a naval vessel Captain François le Clerc had his foot taken off a little above the ankle by a cannon ball. The wound healed but the leg hurt so much that he had it removed five finger-breadths below the knee. Now he could move and walk much better than he could before.

First Use of Ligature in Amputations   (MII,230)

(Paré first reported this method in the Edition of 1564, and had not mentioned it in that of 1552. Presumably, he discovered and used it somewhere in that time period, prob-

---

occupied by Charlemagne's statue. After being destroyed by fire in the 18th century it was rebuilt in its present location on the north side of the island.

Paré left few specific memoirs of his time spent there, but referred proudly on several occasions to the wealth of experience he got.

ably about the time of the Journey to Damvilliers[85] (1552, see pg. 169—ED.)

Galen wrote that it is necessary to tie the vessels toward their roots, which are the liver and the heart, to stanch a great flux of blood. Having used this method of closing the veins and arteries in recent wounds several times in case of hemorrhage, I thought that it could be done also in removal of a limb. I conferred about this with Éstienne de la Rivière, King's Surgeon-in-Ordinary and other Sworn Surgeons of Paris, and on having disclosed my opinion to them, we decided to try it on the first patient who offered himself, keeping the cautery ready for use as did everyone else, in place of a ligature. This I have practiced thus many times with very good results, even a few days ago in the care of Pirou Garbier, a postillion of M. Brusquet, whose right leg was removed four fingers below the knee for a mortification which had developed because of a fracture.

Amputation through Elbow Joint, Tetanus, Recovery   (MII,233)

(A memorable history of the first amputation through a joint in an infected extremity, usually considered fatal in that era—ED.).

I will recount as an example, the history of a cure I performed at Turin in service of M. le Maréschal de Montejan (1538—ED.).

---

[85] A tiny village 15 Km. north of Verdun, which was fortified by Charles V in 1528. On his expedition into this border country of Verdun, Nancy and Metz, Henri II reduced it on July 1, 1552. Here, apparently, Paré first used ligatures to control hemorrhage in amputations.

A poor soldier was shot with an harquebus in the left arm near the wrist and the joint of the hand. The ball lacerated and broke several bones, tendons and other nervous parts. Gangrene developed, then mortification spread nearly to the elbow. Gangrene extended to the shoulder and great inflammation and early gangrene extended to part of the thorax. From this the patient had great belching, excitement and syncope and other severe complications forecasting death. Because the soldier had been abandoned by several Surgeons I was implored by several of his friends to visit him, which I did. After I had seen the mortification, following the precepts of our Art, I was encouraged to remove his arm at the elbow. I did this as rapidly as I could, removing the arm without a saw since the mortification was just beyond the elbow, commencing the amputation by cutting the ligaments joining the bones. This amputation through a joint is not novel, for Hipprocates recommended it in the fourth Section of his book *The Articles,* and said the cure is quick and there is nothing more to fear than fainting from the pain of the incision of the tendons and common ligaments.

My incision made, a great flow of blood followed from the vessels of the part in spite of the tourniquet. I let enough flow to drain and disgorge the part and also to discharge the gangrene in the arm, which encouraged mortification. Then I arrested the blood with the actual cautery, not knowing at the time any other way to accomplish it. This done I loosened the tourniquet gently and made several deep wide incisions in the gangrenous area, avoiding the inner part of the arm because of the great veins, arteries and multitude of nerves that are there. Then I applied the cautery to some of the incisions, as much to arrest the bleeding as to dry up and consume any virulent particles embedded in the part, then applied the dressing mentioned above. On the inflammation of the chest I put large amounts of refrigerants and restrictive medicines and epithemes over the heart. I gave him cordial potions, which I continued until the hiccoughing and other complications arising from the vapors caused by the decay and carried to the heart by the arteries had ceased and desisted.

But I cannot omit to recount (so you may avoid it) that fifteen days later the poor soldier developed a convulsion which I had foretold, because of the cold, since he was poorly housed in a granary where he had only a little cover and was exposed to the wind, without fire and other necessities of human existence. Seeing him in such spasm and contraction of the extremities, the teeth clenched and all the lines of the face drawn and tense, as if he wished to laugh the Sardonic grin, which are manifest signs of convulsion, aroused my pity. Desiring to follow the precepts of my Art, not knowing what else to do, I had them put him in a stable in which was a great number of beasts and a great quantity of manure. Then I managed to have fire in two braziers, near which we rubbed his neck, arms and legs, avoiding the breast areas, with liaments designed to combat the spasms. After wrapping the patient in a warm sheet we put him into the manure in a bed of straw with which we covered him, then covered him with the manure, where he remained three days and nights without arising. Then he had a little bowel movement and a great sweat and began to open his mouth a little. Little by little we aided him with instruments put between his teeth. After opening the mouth with this instrument, I inserted a little wooden rod to keep the mouth open. Since he could not chew, I had them give him milk and egg yolks. By these means were the convulsions cured.

Then followed the cure of the arm, repeating the application of the cautery on the tip of the bone to consume and dry the foreign humors. Worthy of note was the pleasure the patient had when these cauteries were applied, for he said a feeling of tickling ran along the bone from the heat of the cautery carried through the bone. I have seen this several times in the Hôtel-Dieu in Paris in similar cases. Thus great sheets or scales came away from the end of the bone, as much from exposure to air as from the application of the cauteries. I also poulticed the affected part to dry and restore it, which poultices were made with a dry, astringent wine, in which were boiled red roses, absinthe, sage, laurel, flowers of camomile and melilot, anise and other remedies. By such means the poor soldier was healed.

Separation of Callus Around a Fistula (MII,272)

Often the callus around the sinus or cavity of a fistula, the result of sharp and scarring medications, separates and comes away completely leaving the fistula open and bright red. This I have seen in a Gentleman having a fistula of the thigh from a harquebus wound. Having used acrid medications like strong Egyptiac, some days later the eschar came away from the edges of the fistula like a membrane. Seeing it, the Gentleman considered it to be some cloth the Surgeon who had first dressed him had not recognized and taxed him for his carelessness. Realizing it was the crust of the eschar, I told him it was hard, calloused flesh that I had caused to separate by means of strong softening medications. This made him feel better since it was a sign that he soon would be healed. And so it was, because I instilled my balm into the whole cavity.

Suffocation from Too-Tight
Abdominal Binder   (MII,293)

Too tight binding of the abdomen and parts used for breathing can cause suffocation and sudden death. One of recent memory happened in 1581 in the Church of St. Nicholas-des-Champs, when the young wife of Jean de la Forest, Master Barber-Surgeon of Paris, daughter of the late Jacques Ochede, lace merchant and of Claude Boufault, being too bound and compressed in her wedding dress, came from the altar after having taken bread and wine in the accumstomed manner, thinking to return to her place, fell rigidly dead from suffocation. She was buried the same day in the same Church.

And some days later, the said de la Forest married the said Boufault, mother of the dead girl at St. Germain-en-Laye, because his Curé had refused to marry them, saying that one could not espouse the daughter and the mother.

Interrupted Healing, Gunshot
Wound of Scapula   (MII,310)

M. le Marquis de Villars was recently shot in this part (the scapula—ED.) with a pistol at the battle of Dreux[86] (Dec. 19, 1562—ED.) and since then several bone spicules,

---

[86] Dreux—a town of 17,000 inhabitants 35 Km. north of Charters. The battle of Dreux was fought on December 19, 1562 between the Catholics under Guise, the Constable and St. André against the Huguenots under Coligny, Condé and d'Andelot. The Catholics won, but the Constable was wounded and captured and St. André killed. Condé was captured by the Catholics. In 1593 the village was partly burned and the fortress dismantled. Some remains of it are to be seen yet on the grounds of the Chapel of St. Louis, built in 1816 as a necropolis for the Orléans family. This is surrounded by some of the ancient fortifications.

some pieces of his armor and of the ball had been removed. The wound then healed and closed. Later after the battle of Moncontour (1569—Ed.), when he had long worn his armor on his back, a new swelling and inflammation developed in the scar. It opened and several bone spicules and a portion of the bullet came out.

Wounds of Shoulder Joint, Special Dangers   (MII,311)

If the fracture is made at the neck of the shoulder blade or at the shoulder joint, rarely do they recover, however much diligence one can use. This is what happened to the late King of Navarre,[87] to M. de Guise and to Count Ringrave Philebert[88] and several others in these recent battles (of the Civil Wars—Ed.). This is because around this joint are many great vessels, especially the axillary vein and artery and the nerves originating from the cervical

---

[87] Antoine de Bourbon, born in 1518, a brother of Louis, Prince de Condé and of the Cardinal de Bourbon, was duc de Vendôme until he became King of Navarre in 1548 by his marriage to Jeanne d'Albret, the Queen of Navarre. She was a daughter of Queen Margaret of Navarre, favorite sister of King François I. In 1552 he took the rather reluctant Paré into his service and to the siege of Château le Comte, near Hesdin. Paré's good work there caused Antoine to recommend him to King Henri II, who appointed him one of his Surgeons-in-Ordinary in August. The King of Navarre was the "Fifth King" Paré occasionally mentioned serving. Paré attended him on his deathbed following a gunshot wound of the shoulder at the siege of Rouen in 1562. He was interred at the Château Guillard. His son Henri then became King of Navarre and King Henri IV of France in 1590.

[88] Count "Philebert" Ringrave, correctly, Philippe, Jean Philippe II, oldest son of Philippe, François de Dauhn, born in 1545 and cousin by marriage of de Bassompierre. He suffered a shoulder wound at Moncontour similar to that of the King of Navarre at Rouen, and died at the age of twenty-four years.

vertebrae that distribute themselves to all the muscles of
the arm. When inflammation and putrefaction develop,
they are easily transmitted to the heart and other noble
parts, causing many complications and often death.

Fracture of Sternum   (MII,311)

(Malgaigne notes that this history was not in the edition
of 1573, having been added in 1579. The date is wrong, as
the King of Navarre died in 1561. Probably it should read
1553—Ed.).

In 1563 I was sent by the late King of Navarre, King's
Lieutenant-General, to treat Antoine Benand, Lord of
Ville-Neuf, Chevalier of the Order of the King and Gentlemen of his Chamber, Captain of three hundred men, who
was wounded at the Gate of the town of Meun, by a musket
shot in the middle of the sternum. His cuirasse drove in the
bone of the sternum causing him to fall to the ground as if
dead, losing a large quantity of blood by mouth, and he
coughed for three months thereafter. To reduce the bone I
proceeded as I have described and he healed perfectly and
is still living.

Fracture of Neck of Femur   (MII,325)

(Malgaigne notes that this is the first description in medical literature of fracture of the neck of the femur. It first
appeared in the Edition of 1575—Ed.)

Sometimes fracture of the neck of the femur occurs at
the hip joint, which I saw when called to treat a good
woman. Seeing that the leg was shorter than the other, with

a prominence the trochanter makes externally and below the joint of the ischium, I assumed this was the head of the bone, dislocated and not fractured. Then I pulled and set the bone, it seemed, in its socket, after which the two legs were equal in length and contour, and I dressed and treated it as a dislocation. Two days later I found her in great pain, the leg short again and the foot turned inward. I removed the bandages and found that the prominence had reappeared. Then I tried again to replace the bone in its socket and I felt the bone crepitate. Then I found there was no joint cavity, so I knew this was a fracture and not a dislocation.

(Likewise, the epiphysis of the head of this bone sometimes separates and disjoints, so the Surgeon is deceived, thinking it as a dislocation and not disjunction of the epiphysis of this bone.)

Again I reduced the bone, applying splints on the compresses and made a bandage of two parts, crossing them at the joint and around the body like a St. Andrew's cross. The rest of the cure was made as described earlier; I put a hoop over the foot to keep pressure off the toes. I attached a rope to a frame over the middle of the bed, as one should always do in case of fractures of the thigh and leg, to let the patients raise themselves by their arms when they see to their affairs, and also to let them turn a little to lift the back and hips to relieve pressure on the parts, which when denied a long time, produces pain and a strange heat. On this can follow ulceration, most often of the rump, which produces pain, fever and such great upset that death follows, if not well treated. More important than the fracture alone is that near the joints the parts are bloodless and more difficult to treat and harder to cure, because of the nerves, tendons and common ligaments which carry the greatest complications.

A fracture made in the middle of the bone is easier to treat and heals quicker.

Spontaneous Fracture of Painful Joints
(MII,327)

The late M. Marchant, Advocat to the Châtelet of Paris, a man of honor and good doctrine and experience, had a dislocation of the knee joint that tormented him for eight months. He called several learned people, Physicians as well as Surgeons, to relieve him which they could not do by any means because the disease was in the bone. One day he turned in bed and the femur broke near the knee, of which he died soon after. The thigh was opened and was found fractured and the epiphysis separated from the bone, both being carious and purulent, yet he never had had the pox.

Compound Fracture of Leg, Paré's Personal Case
(MII,328)

(In the Edition of 1564 Paré dated this injury on May 4, 1561 and included Antoine Portail in the party, entitling both Portail and Hubert Master Barber-Surgeons—ED.)

To better instruct the young Surgeon I will give a history that was very dear to me.

The misfortune overtook me in the presence of the late M. Nestor,[89] Regent Physician of the Faculty of Medicine and of Richard Hubert, King's Surgeon-in-Ordinary (whose name is well known). We were going to visit some

---

[89] Jean Nestor, born in Paris, received his medical degree on September 24, 1550.

patients at the town of Bons-Hommes,[90] near Paris. On wishing to cross the water, in putting my horse on the boat, I switched him across the rump. The excited beast kicked me, entirely breaking the two bones of the left leg, four fingers above the ankle. Having received the blow and fearing the horse would kick me again, I stepped back a pace, but suddenly fell down. The broken bones came out through the flesh, stocking and boot, from which I felt as much pain as a man can endure.

My bones thus broken and the foot distorted, I feared greatly that it would be necessary to amputate the leg. Turning my eyes and my mind to Heaven, I called my God and prayed Him in His benign grace to help me in my extreme necessity. Immediately I was carried into the boat to cross the river to make my dressing, but the movement almost killed me, as the ends of the bone sawed against the flesh and those who carried me could not help it.

Finally I was carried to a village house with more pain than I had endured in the boat, for one held my body, another the leg, another the foot and in walking one pulled to the left, the other bore to the right. Finally they laid me on a bed to catch by breath and I found my clothing soaked with perspiration from a generalized sweat, and if I had been thrown into the water I would have been no more wet. Then they treated me with such a medication as we could get in such places, composed of egg white, flour and chimney soot with fresh melted butter.

Then I begged M. Richard Hubert not to spare me more than any stranger in his care; that in reducing the fracture, he forget the friendship he bore me. Moreover I admon-

---

[90] The village of Bons-Hommes was the original site of the later Chaillot or Trocadero. The ferry Paré used must have crossed the Seine at about the site of the present Pont d'Iena, in front of the Eiffel Tower.

ished him (even though he knew his Art well) to strongly pull the foot straight and that if the wound was not large enough, to open it with his razor and let him easily put the bones in their normal positions, and that he search the wound carefully with his fingers, which are better than any instrument (for the sense of touch is more certain than any instrument) for removing the fragments and pieces of bone that can be widely separated. Also that he express and force out the blood which was abundant around the wound. He should bandage and place the leg as he knew how to do, in doing this to use three bands as we have described above, and that he start to bandage the wound itself; then splints are added, some three fingers wide, the others two and half-a-foot long and bent to better lie around the leg; they also should be less large at the ends and about a finger width apart. These are tied with little bands of thread like those women tie in their hair. All this is done to the end that the fractured area be supported and held better than otherwise.

After the leg was thus bound, I had them fill the cavity of the knee-joint and that between the saddle of the leg and the ankle with compresses made of flax wrapped in cloth. Then were applied two splints or torches made of straw in which were placed little rods to hold the straw firm and round and enclosed in a half-shroud, then applied to the sides of the leg extending from the heel to the groin, tied in four places to prevent the leg from turning from side to side. And afterward it was put into a straight and not curved position, and raised a little, gently and slowly, to prevent pain, dislocation, inflammation and other accidents.

But it should be noted that if one sets the leg badly, he makes the patient lame, because if the foot is left too high the fracture remains concave in front. Contrarily, if it is left too low, it will be convex or gibbous in front.

Moreover you should observe that if one fails to fill well the concave place between the saddle of the leg and the ankle, the heel will suffer greatly from long pressure which causes great pain (which I know from having felt it myself), because the spirits cannot move well and often they make a strange heat. When hunting the cause of such pain, often I lift the heel a little to give it air so the spirits can flow and some vapor transpire.

And to tell it in a word, my leg was rested on a pillow, banded and tied with struts of straw as you see in the accompanying figure (not reproduced in this book).

Compound Fracture of Leg: Subsequent Treatment of Paré   (MII,334)

To return to my misfortune, my leg was treated point by point as described. I was taken to my house where I was bled of three palettes by the left basilic. At the second dressing and others following, I was cared for by my companions and friends, Sworn Surgeons of Paris. (In the 1564 Edition he said that Étienne de la Rivière took principal charge of him—Ed.)

Rose ointment was applied around the wound and its neighboring parts. This is strongly praised by the ancients for fractures, since it quiets pain and prevents inflammation. It repels humors from the injured part, since it is cold, astringent and repressive. It is made of oil of omphacin, rose water, a little vinegar and white wax. Its use is continued to the sixth day.

The compresses and bands were treated with oxycrat in some coarse astringent wine to strengthen the part. This was especially recommended by Hippocrates for fractures with wounds (compound fractures—Ed.) to dry and drive out the humors. When they are dry, I irrigate them with oxycrat, alternating with oxyrhodinum. For when they are too dry, pain and inflammation return to the part, since they squeeze more when moist. Some Surgeons use only astringent medications and ointments from beginning to end in such a case, unlike the method of Hippocrates and Galen. They consider that with astringents and ointments, they stop the skin pores of the part. This increases the strange heat, with severe pruritis and itching. This engenders under the skin a certain serous, acrid and morbid moisture which makes ulcers. This makes it well to remember not to continue such medications more than five or six days. In place of these one should use ointments described later.

And to return to my story, I was treated from the start of my illness with such an extreme diet that for nine days I ate no more each day than a dozen Damas plums with six morsels of bread and drank a pint of hippocras water (boiled sweetened water flavored with cinnamon—ED.). At other times I had boiled water with syrup *Capil. Vener.* or Divine Drink (boiled sweetened water flavored with lemon—ED.). These are all mixed in glass bottles or other drinking vessels. Sometimes I used a bolus of cassia with a little rhubarb. At other times soap suppositories were used to stimulate the bowel; I dreaded this greatly because when I went some time without a bowel movement, I developed a great heat in the kidneys.

Even such an exquisite regimen could not protect me against the fever that seized me on the eleventh day, with drainage which caused an abscess which suppurated a long time. I believe all of this happened because of some humor retained in the part, as well as not having been able to stand having the wound tightly enough bandaged at first, as well as for some comminuted fragments separated from the ends of the bones, made both by the fracture and its reduction. For the ends were not quite equal and when some little fragments separated, they could not unite and agglutinate. So they changed and decayed, which often is why an abscess and other complications develop.

But the signs that let me know that some bone had separated was that the wound gave out a clear discharge and swelled, while its edges were greatly enlarged and the flesh lax and moist like a sponge. Beyond such causes, it seems to me that the principal occasion of the fever and the abscess came when one night while asleep, the muscles contracted with such great violence that I raised my leg in the air, in such a way that the bones got out of position and pressed the edges of the wound. So it was necessary to pull them out again to reduce them. This hurt even more than when it was first dressed.

This fever continued seven days, at the end of which it terminated partly by drainage and partly by profuse sweating.

(Paré continues here with several pages in which he includes a mixture of explanation of the healing of fractures, advice for treatment and nursing care, with his personal experiences. On page 342 he continues his report—ED.)

It was another month before I could put the foot to the ground without support. This was painful at first, because the callus held the muscles. For, before the movement can be free, it is necessary that the tendons and the membranes become loosened little by little where attached to the scar.

(Malgaigne notes: "The Edition of 1564, and again that of 1575 adds here: 'Finally, thanks to God, I was entirely healed without limping in any way.' " He adds: "It is somewhat astonishing that this essential phrase was omitted in the subsequent editions. In that of 1575 the observation was completed by the two following paragraphs (p. 343) but it was not thus in 1564, which ended with the phrase:

'On which I will conclude the treatment of fractures, praying God that He will protect those who read this history from such complications and especially from death, from which He delivered me; in all things His will be done.' "

By adding the time periods mentioned in the text it is estimated that Paré was back in practice by September, 1562.—ED.)

Anterior Dislocation of Shoulder   (MII,378)

I saw this only once, in the case of a nun who wished to leave her nunnery. She jumped from a window to the ground and falling on the elbow, made an anterior dislocation of the shoulder.

Temporal Arteriotomy for Headache
(MII,411)

I will present the history of M. le Prince de la Roche-sur-Yon,[91] who was extremely tormented by a headache, day and night with little intermission. He called to his treatment Messrs. Chapelain, Premier Surgeon of the King and Castellan, Physician of the Prince and Premier of the Queen-Mother,[92] and M. Duret, Lecturer and Physician-in-Ordinary to the King, very learned men, greatly

---

[91] Charles de Bourbon, second son of Jean II de Bourbon, Prince de la Roche-sur-Yon, married Phillippes de Montespedon, widow of Paré's first Master-at-war, René de Montejan, by whom he had three children. Lieutenant-General of the King's Armies in 1557, Governor of Dauphine in 1562, he died October 10, 1565.

[92] Catherine de' Médicis (1519-1589), daughter of Duke Lorenzo de' Médicis, married the Dauphin Henri (October 8, 1533) during the reign

honored among educated men. They ordered various remedies, external as well as internal, including bleedings, cuppings, baths, massages, in brief, everything they could think of, none of which relieved the pain. Then I was sent for to see if I had any way of stopping the pain. I promptly advised opening the temporal artery on the side of his greatest pain. I told him I had great confidence the cause of his pain was confined to the arteries and not the veins, that I often had made such openings curing the patients and that the ancients advised it. Also I told him that I myself had had it opened for a similar pain and since I had felt no pain. He immediately questioned the Physicians, who agreed with me. In their presence, choosing the artery most noticeable at the temple and which had the strongest pulsation, I opened it with a simple incision, as to make a phlebotomy. I drew two or more palettes of blood, which came out very impetuously, spurting far because of its systole and diastole. I declare that by means of this opening he immediately lost his pain which never returned to him. For this the Prince made me an honorable present.

Exophthalmos (MII,428)

Sometimes by this prominence or prolapse (of the eyes —Ed.) vision is lost, the eye cracks and the humors come out. I actually saw this happen to the sister of Loys de

---

of François I, of whom she was a great favorite. When Henri II became King he neglected her for his favorite, Diane de Poitiers. Upon the King's death, she assumed tremendous power through the successive reigns of her sons, Kings François II, Charles IX and Henri III. Attempting to maintain balance of power between the warring Catholics and Huguenots for the benefit of her sons, she probably unjustly attained an evil reputation for intrigue and murder. She died on January 5, 1589, seven months before Henri III was assassinated, ending the reign of the Valois Kings of France.

Billy, a Merchant Draper living near St. Michel's bridge in Paris. She had such extreme pain, inflammation and discharge that her eyes came out of her head in my presence.

Tooth-ache   (MII,443)

I remember a chamber-varlet of the late M. le Connestable[93] told me when I was in Chantilly, that for an extreme tooth-ache he suffered, had he not feared being damned, he would have jumped out a window into the moat and drowned himself to be rid of the pain. Moreover he told me that in twenty-four hours he had a swelling on the gum, which suppurated at the site of his pain. A few days later the tooth fell apart, which shows that the teeth can abscess and rot like other bones. This one sees because they become pierced and corrode and worms develop in this decay.

---

[93] Anne de Montmorency (1492-1567), made High Constable by François I in 1538. A very important Duke of France, descendent of the "First Christian Barons" and builder of Chantilly; companion-in-arms of Kings François I, Henri II and Charles IX. He was a solid Catholic during the Religious Wars and at the age of seventy-five was in the fray at St. Denis (November 10, 1567) where he received a paralyzing spinal wound. At his wife's request King Charles sent Paré to treat him but the old warrior died in coma a few days later (see p. 190).

Sons:
> François, commanded Therouenne at its fall to Emperor in 1553; became Maréschal after death of his father in 1567. Married Diane de France after death of duc Horace Farnese at Hesdin (1553). Henri, Guillaume, Gabriel and Charles.

Nephews (sons of his sister, Louise de Montmorency):
Odet, Cardinal de Châtillon
Gaspard de Châtillon, Sieur de Coligny, Admiral of France
François de Châtillon, Sieur d' Andelot

Reattachment of Loosened Teeth   (MII,449)

One of my neighbors and friend, Anthoine de la Rue,[93a] Master Tailor of Suits, lived at the end of St. Michel's bridge. He was struck a blow by the pommel of a dagger on his lower mandible so it was completely fractured and three teeth laid reversed in his mouth, nearly out of their sockets. The fracture of the mandible was reduced and the teeth replaced, tied and attached with double waxed thread to their neighbors. I ordered foods for him that did not require chewing, such as juices, gravy, hulled barley, bread-soup, jellies, juice of shoulder of mutton, and other things required by the fracture. Finally he was healed so that to-day he chews as well with these teeth as he ever did.

Pulling Wrong Teeth   (MII,453)

M. François Louis, a Master-Barber of Orléans,[94] had a reputation as a good tooth-puller, so every Saturday several peasants with tooth-ache came to him to have them pulled. This he did very dextrously with a forcep, and when he had used it, he threw it on a shelf in his shop. But he had a new servant, a big strong Picard who wanted to pull teeth as his master did. While François Louis was eating, a villager arrived, requesting that someone pull a

---

[93a] Antoine de la Rue, a tailor and friend who lived near Paré on the Place St. Michel. Pierre de la Rue, probably Antoine's son, married Catherine de Prime, a relative of Ambroise's wife Jeanne Mazelin. Le Paulmier, pg. 35 reprinted an account of Pierre and an accomplice stabbing a teacher named Mercier and throwing him into the river in 1588.

[94] A city of 76,000 people, famous since Roman days; Julius Caesar and Attila have conquered it and Jeanne d'Arc recovered it from the English. Paré was in and out of the place with the Court on numerous occasions, and attended François II here in December, 1560 in his fatal illness.

tooth for him. This Picard took his master's instrument and tried to do as he did, but instead of pulling the poor villager's bad tooth, he pulled three good ones. Feeling much pain and seeing three teeth out of his mouth, he began to cry against the Picard who, to quiet him said he should say nothing and not cry so loud, for if his master heard it, he would make him pay for three teeth instead of one. Now the master, hearing such roaring, left the table to learn the reason for the noise and argument. The poor peasant fearing the threats of the Picard and moreover, after having endured such pain, to have to pay triple the debt to the Picard, he kept quiet not daring to reveal this masterpiece to the Master. And so the poor man strolled back to the village as he had come, and for a tooth he thought to have drawn, he carried away three in his purse and the one causing the pain in his mouth.

Therefore I advise those wishing to have teeth drawn, to go to old dentists and not to young ones who have not yet learned their faults.

Suppression of Urine by Delayed Voiding (MII,498)

Recently a young servant was returning from the field carrying on the rump of his horse a well-accompanied, honest girl, his mistress. While on horseback the need to void seized him, but he could not dismount, nor even less to void on the horse. Arriving in this city and wishing to void, he could not. Having great pains and spasms with a generalized sweat, he almost fainted. I was called to see him and was told they thought a stone prevented him voiding. Having arrived, I put a sound in the bladder and pressed the belly and he passed about a pint of water. I found no stone, and he has not since felt one.

Hematuria from Hard Riding (personal case)
(MII,500)

Those who have been too long on horseback may void blood. This I know myself; going by post to the camp at Perpignan (1542—ED.), near Lyon I pissed pure blood. Really, one ought not to say pissing blood when it comes from the penis pure, but should say passing blood.

Abdominal Wound with Hematuria
(MII,500)

M. Selecgue, a German, Colonel of Mercenaries, received in this city a sword thrust through the belly and incontinently passed blood and fecal matter by penis, bowel and through the wound. He was treated by M. de la Corde, Celebrated Physician in Paris, and M. Pigray, King's Surgeon-in-Ordinary and myself and God healed him. I have seen several who had such wounds and survived, and others with lesser ones who died of them.

Pus in Urine and Stool from Arm Wound
(MII,500)

I saw M. Sarret, King's Secretary, who was shot with a pistol in the right arm. His wound sustained several complications and abscesses, from which drained a large quantity of pus and for several days only a little drained. And then he passed it by bowel and by his urine, and when the ulcers drained a great deal, one did not see in the stool or urine any sign of pus. He was cured, thanks to God, and is still living.

Arm Wound with Purulent Drainage by Stool and Urine   (MII,500)

M. Houlier, Regent Physician of the Faculty of Medicine of Paris, Germain Cheval and M. (François) Rasse, Sworn Surgeons, excellent Medical men, and I treated M. de la Croix, a Gentleman who was wounded by a sword thrust in the left arm, to whom a similar thing happened, but he died.

But M. Rasse said it was impossible for pus to take so long a route to be evacuated, adding that it could not go by the veins unless mixed with the blood and therefore it could rather come from the mesentery or intestines and not from the arm or such other part. I said on the contrary that it came from the arm because when the ulcers drained freely it did not drain from below. M. Houlier was on my side saying the ancients had left in writing that such things could be. What could put us in agreement would be to seek in his body, if he should die, to see if he had an ulcer or abscess.

He died and the body was opened in our presence. After examining all the internal parts, no place was found where the pus could drain. So it was concluded that the pus came from the arm and was discharged by stool and urine; ending that such is not impossible because our bodies are flexible and transpirable.

Diabetes, Strangury and Bladder Ulcers   (MII,510)

I remember treating with M. Houlier, a learned Doctor, the late M. Goyet, King's Advocat at the Châtelet of Paris, who had difficulty retaining his urine, called strangury, and voided as much during the day as at night, with great pain.

He complained of great heat and burning in the bladder and at the end of the penis. He passed milky urine and at the end of urination, pus. We gave him many remedies and to ease his pain, on M. Houlier's advice, I gave him injections with plantain water and centinodium in which was dissolved chalk and bole. At other times I injected mucilages of quince and psyllium with water of plantain and rose, which remedies tended finally to refresh the heat of the bladder and dry the ulcers.

Discussing with Houlier to know the cause of such complications, I said Goyet had a rough and contracted bladder with little ulcers, and when the urine fell in the bladder it irritated it, which made it want to eject it promptly. The pus that flowed after the urine came from the ulcers in the bladder from the compression it made to pass the urine.

The said Goyet having died, I opened his body in the presence of M. Houlier and we found the bladder all callused and full of pustules the size of small peas; when I compressed these white pus drained, such as was passed with the urine during his life.

Fecal Retention—Cause of Death (MII,515)

I remember having opened the dead body of a twelve year old boy, who had all his intestines entirely filled with very hard, dry fecal matter. Before death he passed this by mouth, which was the cause of his death, failure to get help at a suitable time.

Colic, Cured by Passing Bullet (MII,519)

M. Jean de St. Germain, an accomplished Parisian Apothecary swore to me he had treated a gentleman having the colic, with extreme pain. To help himself he had taken several clysters and other things ordered by learned Physicians, but his pain continued. A German friend advised him to drink three ounces of cold-pressed oil of almonds mixed with white wine and parietary water. He did this, then they had him swallow a lead harquebus ball shined and whitened with quick-silver (so it would go down better). Soon afterward he passed it by stool and immediately his pain stopped.

Family Infected with Syphilis by Baby's Nurse (MII,529)

An honest, rich wife begged her husband to let her nurse her baby. He permitted this, provided she take another nurse to help her nourish the infant. This nurse had the pox and gave it to the infant, the infant to the mother, she to her husband and the husband to the two other children with whom he ordinarily ate and drank. They often slept with him, not knowing that he was infected with this disease. But the mother saw the baby was not gaining and cried constantly. She sent for me to know the cause of the illness, which was not hard to tell, since the baby was covered with pimples and ulcers; the nipples of the nurse were ulcerated, as were those of the mother. She had pimples on her body, as did the husband and the two small children, three and four years old. Then I told the father and mother that they had syphilis, brought to them by the nurse. I treated them and they recovered, except the little baby, who died. The nurse was lashed in prison and would have had it in the streets had it not been for fear of dishonoring the house.

Suppression of Urine-Prostatitis-Autopsy
(MII,559)

There was a man who after violent excesses was taken with a suppression of urine so he could not urinate without the help of a sound he always carried with him. One day he could not get it into the bladder and sent for me to make him void. This I could not do, although I used all the remedies possible, which was the cause of his death.

This having happened, I asked his wife to let me open him, which she granted me. I found his bladder full of urine and greatly stretched. The prostrate was swollen, ulcerated and full of pus like that he passed during his illness.

Stinking Feet   (MII,601)

I remember treating a Prince of some malady and the Apothecary's servant had such stinking feet that one smelled them when he entered the room. He knew they smelled and to remedy it he rubbed the soles of his feet with a great deal of musk. Instead of stopping and lessening the odor, it augmented it so that he perfumed the room he entered with an odor so strong and stinking that one could not endure it. This caused him to be discharged and banished from the Prince's house.

Plastic Reconstruction of the Nose
(MII,606)

We have information of this (plastic reconstruction of nose) from a young Gentleman, the Cadet of St. Thoan, who had lost his nose and for a long time wore a silver one, taking offense at remarks made without a laugh when he was in company. Having been told there was a Master re-builder of noses in Italy, he went to find him. He rebuilt one for him as described above, as many people have seen since, not without the great admiration of those who had known how he looked with a nose made of silver.

Appliance to Assist Speech in Absence of Tongue (MII,608)

A certain individual living at the town of Yuoy-le-Châ-teau, ten to twelve leagues from Bourges, had a part of his tongue cut off and lived three years unable to have his speech understood. It happened that he was in the fields with some reapers drinking from a thin wooden dish. One of them tickled him as he had the dish between his teeth and he uttered words that could be understood. Immedi-ately realizing he had spoken thus, he took the dish and replaced it in the same position and spoke again, under-standably. For a long time he carried it in his bosom to help him talk, always putting it between his teeth.

Sometime later he had made (by necessity, which is the Mother of Arts) a wooden instrument, as the figure shows which he carried hanging from his neck. By this means he was able to make understood by speech all that he wished to say. (Figure not reproduced in this book.)

Speech Appliance, for Loss of Tongue (MII,609)

I was shown this instrument and its manner of use by the wise Physician, M. le Tellier[95] of Bourges. I knew a young lad whose tongue was cut off. Thanks to the use of this

---

[95] Durand le Tellier, a Bourges physician who later served King Henri IV, being succeeded in 1606 by his son Simon.

instrument he trained his speech so well that one could understand everything he wanted to say. With this proof, everyone can do the same when confronted with this problem.

Appliance for Extending Thumb   (MII,613)

When nerve or tendon is entirely severed the action they produce is lost and the part remains unable to flex or extend, which may be aided by the artifice of the surgeon.

That is what I did for one of M. le Connestable's Gentlemen who received a cutlass stroke the day of the battle of Dreux (Dec. 19, 1562—ED.) near the joint of the right hand, on the back, cutting the tendons raising the thumb. After healing, the thumb remained flexed in his hand, so he could not open it without the help of the other hand, after which it immediately flexed again as before. Because of this, the Gentleman could not hold sword, dagger, lance, pike nor other arms. Seeing his hand thus useless and deprived of weapons, he begged me to cut off his thumb. I did not want to do this to him, but made for him an instrument of tin in which to put his thumb. This instrument was attached by two lanyards to two little rings on the joint of the hand so dextrously that the thumb remained raised. Thus the Gentleman could grasp sword, pike, lance and other arms. This figure shows it (not reproduced in this book).

Extraction of Dead Foetus   (MII,629)

I was called once to deliver from the mother a dead infant which the midwives, so-called sage women, had tried to withdraw by one of its arms, which had caused gangrene and mortification of the arm and the death of the infant. They could not replace the arm because of the swelling of

the mother's genitals and of the baby's arm. It was necessary to remove and amputate it.

The way to do this is to cut it with the razor as near the
shoulder as possible, always observing in making the incision, to draw the fleshy parts up, then cut the bone with
proper forceps, so that flesh will cover the end of the bone
so it will not injure the uterus and other genital parts. That
done, find the feet of the infant and pull them down if
possible as described earlier, etc.

Separation of Pubis in Labor. Autopsy (MII,668)

But what made me hold this idea is that which I have
maintained by word and by writing, the pubic bone cannot
separate and open any at delivery. Nevertheless the contrary was demonstrated to me on Feb. 1, 1579 by the dissection of a women who died fifteen days after having
been delivered. I saw the dissection and found the pubic
bone separated in its center about one half inch, in the
presence of M. Claude Rebours,[96] Regent Physician of the
Faculty of Medicine, M. Jean d'Amboise,[97] Cointeret, du
Bois,[98] Dionneau,[99] Larbalestrier and Viard,[100] all Sworn

---

[96] Rebours received his medical degree in 1572. He was a member of
the Faculty Commissions appointed to pass upon the publication of the
second edition of Paré's "Oeuvres" in 1578 and the Latin Edition in 1581.

[97] Surgeon of Charles IX and of Henri III. He witnessed the autopsy
done on Charles IX by Paré on May 31, 1574. He had been surgeon of
the Châtelet in 1560, giving up the post voluntarily in 1566 to Robert
Gaignat.

[98] Guillaume du Bois, Surgeon-in-Ordinary to Henri II. He was an
official in the College of Surgeons at Paré's induction in 1554, and was
present when Parè embalmed Charles IX.

[99] Dionneau (Dioniau), Jacques, Sworn Surgeon of Paris, witness of
autopsy of King Charles IX, done by Paré on May 31, 1574.

[100] Claude Viart (frequently spelled Viard by Paré) was a Surgeon of

Surgeons of Paris. We all saw the ischium separated from the sacrum. Who does not want to believe it, I refer to the book of Nature, who does things intelligence is not capable of understanding. And primarily, these bones open and close at delivery.

Hydatid Mole—Autopsy, Mme. Roger (MII,724)

The wife of Guillaume Roger, Master Pewterer in rue St. Victor, aged fifty or more, had carried a mole seventeen years or more. She died on July 27, 1574. Her husband called me to open her body, where I found her uterus had no attachment except its neck and a little omentum. There was only one ovary on the right, quite large, soft and loose. And as for the tubes, there were none apparent, except a little on the same side. There were no vessels except those of the cervix, which were large and superficial. The uterus was as large as the head of a large, powerful man. Having removed it, I took it to my house to dissect it and see what it contained. I did not want to do this without having the company of learned Physicians and Surgeons. These were: M. de Mazille,[101] Counciller and Pre-

---

Nantes who practiced near Paré in Paris. On March 27, 1577 he married Jeanne Paré, Ambroise's favorite niece, daughter of his dead brother Jean, the cabinet maker. Jeanne lived with the Parés after her father's death. Ambroise gave the Viarts one of his group of houses with access to the Place St. Michel. Viart practiced with Paré and died between 1582 and 1584. In 1588 Jeanne remarried with François Foret.

[101] A native of Beauvoisis, Mazille took his degree at Montpellier in 1539, practiced at Beauvais and became Physician of François, duc d'Alencon, younger brother of King Charles IX, of François II, First Physician of Charles IX and Physician-in-Ordinary of Henri III. Le Paulmier (p. 191) recounted conflicting stories about him, that the Queen-Mother wanted to hang him for his favorable prognosis in the

mier Physician of the King, M. Alexis, Premier Physician of the Queen, M. Fibor, Premier Physician of the Queen-Mother, M. de St. Point, Premier Physician of the Queen of Navarre, Messers. le Fèvre,[102] Brouet, King's Physician-in-Ordinary, Messrs. Violaines, Greaume, Marescot, Rauin, Milot, Hautin, Riolan and Lusson,[103] Regent Physicians of the Faculty of Medicine, Cointeret, King's Surgeon to the Châtelet of Paris and Premier of the Queen, le Brun and Guillemeau, Sworn Surgeons of Paris. In their presence I opened the uterus which we found scirrhous and so extremely hard the knife could hardly cut it; the tunic under the peritoneum was otherwise sound and complete. The uterus was three inches or more thick. Within was found flesh resembling a cow's udder, as large as two fists. It was not adherent to the walls except that at certain points it was very dense and lumpy, in the substance of which were infiltrated strange bodies, like atheromes, cartilages and bones. It was the conclusion of all that the origin of this flesh had been a mole, taking nourishment and growing like the wens that develop in some parts of our bodies, which with time become scirrhous and resemble the substance of the uterus. Moreover we found a tumor in the center of the cervix as large and round as a turkey's egg, as hard

---

last illness of Charles IX, but this is discounted by his later appointment by Henri III.

[102] Pierre le Fèvre (Lefèvre) was Physician-in-Ordinary of Kings Charles IX and Henri III and of Catherine de' Médicis. He and Paré consulted on many cases in the Court, and he witnessed Parè's autopsy of King Charles IX.

[103] Lusson was born at Liseux, became a physician in Paris in 1573 and Dean of the Faculty in 1594 to 1595. Lusson was Paré's intermediary for presentation of his Oeuvres (2nd Edition) before the Faculty for their approval prior to its publication. He later became Physician-in-Ordinary of Henri IV and of the Princess de Condé (Le Paulmier, p. 99).

throughout as cartilage and bone. It occupied mainly the internal os of the uterus, vulgarly called the cap, so nothing could enter or leave. The whole weighed nine pounds, two ounces. I kept it in my cabinet as a museum piece.

Hydatid Mole, Case Report—Mme. Roger (MII,725)

While the woman lived she had severe pain in her abdomen which was hard and marvelously large, as if she carried several infants. Several Physicians seeing her pass the normal time for delivery, had treated it as dropsy, but nothing could stop the enlargement of her belly. She also had suppression of urine for two or three days and then voided only with great pain. Meanwhile she would sometimes go seven or eight days without going to stool because of the intestinal compression made by this enormous mass. At intervals of about three months she had great hemorrhages, which could not come out of the cavity of the uterus, since as we have said, it was filled and completely closed, sealed and stopped. But such bleeding occurred from the vessels by which virgins and pregnant women menstruate. To show the remarkable size of this mole I have presented it here in the figure, intact in the first and in the other opened.

Hydatid Mole, Autopsy (MII,727)

I remember having opened the body of a woman who died because she had a mole the size of a goose egg, which Nature wished to cast out and could not; it remained and putrefied, from which death followed.

Uterine Prolapse (MII,740)

I attest having seen and treated a young woman whose uterus descended the size of a large egg, to have been cured and since borne children. Her uterus never fell again.

Vaginal Hysterectomy (MII,745)

A young woman, twenty-five or thirty years old, healthy and well regulated menstrually as she described it, and reputed honest and happy, married a second time in 1571, not having had children by the first marriage. A little later she had signs of conception, but with passage of time felt a disagreeable heaviness in the perineum, with pain, retention of urine and other complications she could not endure. She showed it to her neighbor and friend, Christofle Mombeau, a Barber-Surgeon in the Faubourgs St. Germain-des-Prés. As he reported to me, he saw a swelling of the perineum, and following the custom of his art, applied poultices and plasters of decoctions of herbs and other soothing and emollient remedies, after which the pain ceased. But at the labium minora appeared an opening like an abscess from which for a long time drained pus that was orange, yellow and sometimes livid. Afterwards the heaviness did not abate but increased to the point that between 1573 and the years following to the day of the fall, if the patient wished to turn in bed she could do it easily only by putting her hand on the side of the belly to which she wished to turn. And then she felt as if a lead ball fell to the side to which her body turned. Reclining or seated, she could not void or move her bowels without lifting this weight toward her diaphragm with her hands. Walking, she moved her legs difficultly and always felt something between them that blocked her. Sometime later the opening drained matter and she had pain in the head and other members, failure of the heart, anorrhexia, vomiting and suffocations. Overcome by illness and impatience, on December 27th last, under promise of certain and assured relief, she was persuaded by a female empiric to take antimony. The violence of this was such that after having vomited several times with great effort and made several watery stools, she thought she felt her rectum prolapse. Visited by an old friend, she was advised to call in the Surgeons, for what protruded did not seem to be the rectum, but something else resembling it. I was called the sixth day of January, 1575 and M. Jacques Guillemeau, Sworn-Surgeon of Paris, M. Antoine de Vieux, Master Barber-Surgeon of Faubourg St. Germain-des-Prés, saw her with me.

After having considered everything, we advised that to help her, it was necessary to remove what presented, since it was black, putrid and had other signs of a purulent substance. Se we began to draw painlessly, little by little on alternate days, a body that was judged by Messrs. Alexis Gaudin,[104] Physician-in-Ordinary of the King, and Premier of the Queen, P. le Fèvre, also Physician-in-Ordinary of the King and of Madam le Princess de la Roche-sur-Yon,[105] de Violanes, Doctor in the University of Paris and us Surgeons, to be the body of the uterus, since one of the ovaries was found and a gross membrane remaining from a mole which had abscessed, ruptured and expelled, as the saying is.

---

[104] Alexis Gaudin, Physician of Kings Charles IX and Henri III, and First-Physician of Queens Elizabeth of Austria and Louise de Lorraine.

[105] Princess de la Roche-sur-Yon, Philippes de Montespedon, duchess of Beaupreau, widow of duc de Montejan, later married the Prince de la Roche-sur-Yon. Apparently her friendship for Paré persisted from their Piedmont days and she was godmother to Paré's son Ambroise, baptized on May 30, 1576. The child died in infancy.

After the removal of this part the patient improved. For nine days before the extirpation she had not moved her bowels and for four days had not voided, as she did regularly thereafter. She was well for three months, after which she developed pleurisy, with continuous high fever of which she died.

Autopsy: Being notified she had died, desiring to know what Nature had built in place of the uterus, we opened her. We found no uterus, but in its place was a hard scar Nature had made during the brief three months that remained to try to replace what had been lost.

(In an attack on Paré later, Compèrat claimed that the autopsy showed the uterus to be intact and named two witnesses. Malgaigne said that the facts are impossible to determine. Packard said it was not possible that Paré was the liar!—ED.)

Hymen, Section of   (MII,747)

I had searched many dead girls, aged three, four, five to twelve years, at the Hôtel-Dieu in Paris (for a hymen—ED.), and never found one. Then a seventeen year old girl, engaged for marriage was brought by her mother who knew she had something which could keep her from conceiving. She asked me to see her and I found her to have a nervous membrane as thick as thin parchment between the labia, immediately below the urethra, before the entrance of the vagina, having a little hole through which she could menstruate. Seeing the thinness of the membrane, I cut it promptly with scissors and told the mother how to complete the cure. I charged her expressly to put between the two parts a pledget of lint like a tent, to prevent the union of what had been cut to replace it with another. Later she was married and had children.

Subdural Empyema after Pneumonia
(MII,776)

Mlle. de Chalenge of Brittany having white menses, came to Paris to get medical advice and be cured of this flux, hoping later to have children. But several days later she developed great pain in her side with fever. Doctors le Grand, Duret and Rebours were called; they concluded she had pleurisy with peripneumonia. At that time she had her menses, nevertheless they ordered a clyster and bleeding; she flatly refused. The next day, which was the seventh day of complications, she was bled. M. Duret saw her twice that day and said that if she developed pain and itching of the head, she would die because of passage of material from the lungs to the head. The next day the pain and itching of the head developed and she died a few hours later.

Four or five days later, Drs. Rebours, Viard and I made an autopsy of a priest who died of pleurisy and peripneumonia with headache. We wished to see if the above prognosis held and if material from the lung had gone to the brain. After opening the head, we found the space between the pia-mater and the brain all filled with pus, as in the girl mentioned above.

Pruritis Vulvae   (MII,790)

Recently a women being vexed with this malady (pruritis vulvae—Ed.) asked me to prescribe a treatment and told me she often was obliged to put ashes from the hearth on it to stop the itching. I recommended that she make injections of Egyptiac dissolved in sea water and at other times in lye water. She should also apply pessaries or large tents made of compresses soaked in these liquids. By these means she was cured, after some days.

Umbilical Hernia of Infants   (MII,795)

I have seen this (umbilical hernia—ED.) several times, notably in a baby of the late M. de Martigues. He had married Madame de Laval,[106] who was of the house of Lautrec. Their Surgeon M. Pierre de la Roque was in great personal danger and but for the help of M. d'Estampes and M. de Martigues, the servants would have cut his throat, thinking the child's death the fault of the Surgeon.

Umbilical Hernia of Infants   (MII,795)

And again not long ago, such a thing happened to the infant of Jean de Gourmont, a sculptor living at the Arbre Sec, rue St. Jean de Latran in the University of Paris. He sent for me to inquire about opening the umbilicus. I refused, saying the child would die easier without me. Three days later the abscess ruptured spontaneously and the intestines came out, of which he died.

Failure of Dentition   (MII,799)

M. de Nemours[107] asked me to autopsy his dead eight months old son, who had not erupted any teeth. Having

---

[106] Originally Claude de Foix, she married Guy XVII, Comte de Laval, who with de Rohan had taken Paré to the defense of Landerneau in 1543. Laval died on May 25, 1547 without children. His widow then married M. de Martiques, whose fatal chest wound Paré treated after the fall of Hesdin on July 17, 1553 (Le Paulmier p. 26).

[107] Jacques de Savoy, duc de Nemours, son of Philippe de Savoie, born October 12, 1531 in Champagne. After the death of François, duc de Guise in 1563, he married Guise's widow, Anne d'Este, then thirty-five years old. She was the mother of Henri, who became duc de Guise, and had several children by de Nemours.

carefully sought the cause of his death without finding anything except that the gums were very hard and swollen, I cut through them and found all the teeth ready to erupt, with a little help that might have come from incising the gums. The Doctors present and I concluded that the only cause of death was that Nature had not been strong enough to pierce the gums and push the teeth out. This was because at his age the gums were harder than those of an old person.

Monster: Two-Headed Infant (MIII,8)

In Paris in 1546 a woman six months pregnant gave birth to an infant having two heads, two arms and four legs. I opened it and found only one heart. One can say then that this was a single infant. This monster is in my house, kept as a museum piece.

Monster: Single-Headed Twins (MIII,9)

In 1569 a woman of Tours bore twins having a single head which they shared between themselves. This was given one day and dissected by M. René Ciret, Master Barber-Surgeon whose renown throughout Touraine is great enough without my giving other praise.

The duc had figured in a Court scandal in 1557. Françoise de Rohan, daughter of Paré's old Chief, René de Rohan, had been seduced by the duc under promise of marriage, then abandoned because of Anne d'Este, who was not yet a widow. She sued him and Paré testified at the trial, which she lost on August 10, 1559. The duchess de Nemours was godmother of Paré's daughter Anne on July 16, 1575 and her eight year old son Charles was godfather.

Change of Sex   (MIII,19)

In the suite of the King Charles (IX—ED.) at Vitry-le-François in Champagne (in the tour of the Court around France, 1564—ED.) I saw a certain person named Germain Garnier. Others called him Germain Marie because when a girl he was called Marie. He was a young man of medium height, well proportioned, wearing a thick red beard. Until fifteen years old he had been considered a girl, since he showed no signs of virility, associated with girls and wore their clothes. As he was in the fields vigorously chasing some pigs going into the grain, he found a ditch before him. He jumped and instantly developed the genitals and a virile penis, having broken some ligaments that apparently had kept them enclosed and hidden (this caused him no pain). He returned crying to his mother's house, saying his entrails were coming out of his belly; she was greatly astonished at the spectacle.

Having assembled Physicians and Surgeons to advise her, they found that she was a man and not a girl. They reported it to the Bishop who was the late Cardinal de Lenoncourt. By his authority, at an assembly of the people, he was certified a man and instead of Marie, he was called Germain. He took the dress of a man and I believe he and his mother are still living (in 1579—ED.).

Boy with Deformed Extremities   (MIII,21)

In 1573 I saw at Paris at the door of St. André-des-Arts, a nine year old child born at Parpeuille, a village three leagues from Guise. His father was Pierre Renard, his mother was called Marquette. This monster had only two fingers in the right hand and the arm was well formed from shoulder to elbow, but below the elbow to the two digits, was very deformed. He had no legs, yet from the right buttock grew an incomplete sort of a foot having four toes. From the left buttock grew two toes, one of which somewhat resembling a penis. I show the truth of this in this figure (not reproduced in this book).

Armless Man   (MIII,22)

Until recently one could see in Paris a strong, robust man without arms, about forty years old. He could do almost everything others could do with their hands. With the stump of his shoulder and his head he could chop wood with an ax as well as another man could do with his arms. He could crack a coachman's whip and do many other things. With his feet he ate, drank and played cards and dice, as shown in the figure. Finally he became a scoundrel, thief and murderer and was executed in Gueldre, being hanged and put on the wheel.

Armless Seamstress   (MIII,23)

Similarly, not long ago one could see in Paris a woman without arms, who could sew and cut and do several other things.

Needle Passing Through Thigh   (MIII,29)

Catherine Parlan, wife of Guillaume Guerrier, an honest drapery merchant living on rue de la Juifuerie in Paris, going to the fields on a horse, had a needle from her pincushion enter her right buttock so she could not remove it. For two months she could not sit because she felt the needle piercing. Four months later she sent for me to treat her, complaining that when her husband embraced her, she felt a great pricking pain in the right groin when he pressed down. Putting a hand on the pain, I found a sharp hardness and brought out the needle all rusted. This should be put in the list of monstrous things, since the steel, which is heavy, rose upward and passed through the thigh muscles without producing an abscess.

Bladder Stone Containing Needle   (MIII,29)

In 1566, the sons of M. Laurens Colo, men very experienced in extracting stones, removed one the size of a nut in the middle of which was found a needle with which seamstresses usually sew. The patient, Pierre Cocquin, lived at the Place Mauberg in Paris and is still living. The stone was presented to the King in my presence with the needle, which the Collos gave me to put in my museum, which I keep and still have in my possession to remember such a remarkable thing.

Bladder Stones of M. Tire-vit   (MIII,30)

In 1566, Laurens, brother of Jean Colo, extracted three stones from the bladder. Each was the size of a large hens egg, of white color, weighing three ounces and more, from one called Tire-vit, living at Marly. Since the age of ten years he had some signs of bladder stones causing him to tug at his penis, hence the name "Tire-vit." The expulsive force of the bladder, as of all the body, tries to throw out what irritates it. From this a certain itching occurs at the tip of the penis, as happens ordinarily to those having gravel or stones in parts devoted to urine, as I have written more fully in my book, "Of Stones."

These were presented to the King, then at St. Mauer-des-Fosses. One was broken with a hammer and within it was found another tan one, resembling a peach stone. The Collos gave me these stones to keep in my museum and I had them portrayed in life size, as you can see in the figures (not reproduced in this book).

(See presentation on pg. 4. It is uncertain if two separate incidents were erroneously attributed to the unfortunate Tire-vit, or if he actually had two operations—ED.)

Kidney Stones, Bizarre Forms   (MIII,31)

Moreover, I have found in the kidneys of dead bodies stones of many shapes, such as pigs, dogs and other strange figures, as have been left to us in the writings of the ancients.

Stone in Knee   (MIII,32)

In 1558, I was called by Jean Bourlier, Master Tailor of St. Honoré, to open an aqueous tumor of the knee. In it was found a stone the size of an almond, very white, hard and polished. He recovered and lives at present.

(Malgaigne says this is the first reported case of removal of a foreign body developing in the knee—ED.)

Stone in Bowel   (MIII,32)

A lady of our Court was very ill for a long time, feeling pain in the belly, with great spasms. She was treated by several Doctors who could not find the cause of the pain. I was called to see if I could discover the cause of her illness. By the order of the Physicians I examined the rectum and the uterus with proper instruments and for all that could not discover her lesion. M. le Grand ordered a clyster and in returning it, she passed a stone by rectum. It was as large as a big nut and at once all her pain and complications cleared and she has been well since.

Salivary Calculus   (MIII,32)

Captain Augustin, King's Engineer, called me to treat him with M. Violaine, Regent Physician in the Faculty of Medicine and Claude Viard, Sworn-Surgeon of Paris, to extract a stone he had under his tongue, half an inch long and large as a pen quill. He had another also, which could not easily be detached.

Infant Swallowing Piece of Steel, Autopsy (MIII,40)

The twenty month old baby of de-Pleurs, Drapery Merchant, living at the corner of the new rue Nôtre-Dame of Paris, swallowed a piece of a steel mirror, which descended to the scrotum and caused his death. The body was opened in the presence of M. le Gros, Regent Physician of the Faculty of Medicine of Paris by M. Balthazar, then Surgeon of the Hôtel Dieu. Curious of the truth, I went to talk to Madame de-Pleurs who declared the thing true and showed me the piece of mirror which she carried in her purse.

Vomited Worms   (MIII,40)

In October, 1578, Tiennette Chartier, a forty year old widow living at St. Maur-les-Fosses being ill of a tertian fever, vomited a large quantity of bilious fluid at the onset function

of an attack. With it she ejected three hairy worms, resembling caterpillars in shape, color, length and thickness, except they were darker. They lived eight days or more without any nourishment. They were brought here by the Barber of St. Maur to M. Milot, Physician and Lecturer of the Medical School who was treating the patient and who showed them to me. Doctors le Fèvre, le Gros, Marescot and Courtin[108] also saw them.

Toad in Stone (MIII,43)

In my vineyard near the village of Meudon[109] where I was having some large solid rocks broken, a big, live toad was found in the center of one without any apparent opening. I marvelled how this animal had been born, grew and had life. Then the quarryman told me it was not necessary to marvel, because several times he had found such and other animals in the depth of stone, without any sign of opening. One can explain the birth and life of such animals: they are engendered of some moist substance of stones, which petrified moisture produces such beasts.

---

[108] Germain Courtin graduated in Medicine on July 10, 1576, was named Professor in 1578, teaching surgery with distinction.

[109] A village about five miles from Paré's town houses in Paris, a little off the road to Versailles. In 1550 Paré got a house in Meudon from a brother-in-law in payment of a debt, and kept it as a summer place. In 1551 and 1552, Rabelais was Curé of Meudon, but neither he nor Paré wrote of the other. His old house, which has just been torn down, was on the rue de Pierres, next door to the present town museum. On top of the hill above his house is a splendid Terrasse that overlooks Paris, and upon which the Germans had a gun emplacement in 1871. In his day there was a splendid palace there, built for Anne de Pisseleau, Mistress of François I, sold to the Cardinal de Lorraine, and enlarged by succeeding rulers until the Revolution. Used then as an arsenal, it was so badly damaged by fire, it was torn down in 1805. The Terrasse remains and at one end is an astronomical observatory.

Beggar with Stolen Arm   (MIII,46)

In 1525 I was in Angers,[110] when a wicked knave had cut the purulent and infected arm from a hanged man and fastened it to his doublet, held with a cord against his side. Hiding his good arm behind his back covered with his cloak, he pretended the arm of the hanged man was his. He cried at the door of the temple that one give him alms in honor of St. Anthony. On the day of Holy Friday, all seeing the decayed arm gave him alms, thinking it true. The beggar having removed his arm long since, it detached itself and fell to the ground where all saw it. He was found to have two good arms besides that of the hanged. Then he was taken prisoner, condemned by the order of the Magistrate to be whipped with the decayed arm hanging from his neck in front of his stomach and was banished from the country.

Beggar Feigning Cancer of Breast (MIII,46)

My brother Jehan Paré,[111] a Surgeon in the Brittany town of Vitré, saw a big, plump beggar woman asking alms at the door of a temple one Sunday. She pretended having a cancer of the breast, which was a hideous thing to see because of a great drainage of pus defiling a cloth she had over

---

[110] A town on the river Loire, about 80 Km. south of Paré's birthplace, Laval. Ambroise was there in 1525, at the age of fifteen and witnessed the unmasking of a malingerer. Interestingly, David of Angers was the sculptor who executed the statue of Paré erected in the town square of Laval.

[111] Ambroise's older brother, a Barber-Surgeon of Vitré. It is not known if Ambroise got part of his training with him, as tradition runs; he simply recounts having been with him, observing his detection of malingerers.

it. My brother noticed that her face had good color, showing her to be healthy, and that the parts around the cancerous ulcers were white and of good color, and the rest of her body well nourished. Thinking to himself that this slut could not have a cancer and be so plump, chubby and shiftless, he concluded she was an imposter. He denounced her to the magistrate, called l'Aloüé in that country, who let him take her to his house to prove the deception. When there, he uncovered her breast and found that she had under her armpit a sponge filled with a mixture of animal blood and milk and a little tube of elder by which the mixture was conveyed to the false holes of her cancerous ulcer concealed under the cloth she had over it. Thus he knew the ulcer was artificial. He soaked the breast with warm water and lifted several black, green and yellow frog skins and mixtures of them, glued on with a mixture of paste and egg white, as they found by her confession. Having removed these, the breast was found as healthy as the other. The imposture proved, the Aloüé took her prisoner. She was questioned and confessed saying this was done by the beggar she lived with. He also feigned having an enormous ulcer of the leg, making this appear real by means of a beef spleen he put on and around his leg, applied and fastened appropriately with clever drapes at each end, so it appeared twice normal size. To make the thing more monstrous and hideous to see, he made several cavities in the spleen through which he cast a mixture of blood and milk under its coverings. The Aloüé hunted this master beggar, thief and imposter, but not finding him, condemned her to be put to the whip and banished from the country. She was well lashed with blows of a whip of knotted cords, as they did at that time.

Beggar Feigning Leprosy   (MIII,47)

A year later a great scoundrel came pretending to have leprosy. He put himself at the door of a temple displaying his advertisement. This was a kerchief on which he put his tub and several small pieces of money. In his right hand he had clackers, with which he made a loud clicking noise. His face was covered with big pimples made of strong glue and painted with rouge and livid color, resembling the color of lepers. He was very hideous, so from compassion everyone gave him alms.

My brother (Jehan—ED.) approached him and asked how long he had been sick. He responded in a thick, hoarse voice that he was a leper from birth and that his father and mother had died, their bodies falling apart piece-meal. This leper had a scarf wrapped around his neck and with his left hand under his cloak, he squeezed his throat, causing the blood to rise to his face, making it even more hideous and disfigured. Thus he also made his voice hoarse by constricting his trachea, already bound by the scarf.

My brother continued to chat with him and he could not avoid loosening his scarf to get his breath a little. My brother noticed this and suspected this was some imposter's trick. He went to the Magistrate asking permission to examine him to know the truth. This was granted, ordering him to take him to his house to prove if he was a leper. He first made him take the scarf off his neck, then made him wash his face with hot water. This removed the pimples and his face became clean and natural, without a blemish. This done, he was stripped and his body showed no sign of leprosy. Being informed of this the Magistrate took him prisoner and he was interrogated three days later. He confessed the truth, since he could not deny it, after a long remonstrance by the Magistrate showing him to be a public thief, being healthy and fit to work. The leper told him he knew no other trade than counterfeiting the ills of St. John, St. Fiacre and St. Main. In brief, he could counterfeit several maladies, but none was more remunerative than feigned leprosy. Then he was condemned to be whipped through the streets on three successive Sundays with his tub hanging from his neck on his chest and his clackers behind his back, then banished forever from the country under threat of the rope.

When the last Sunday came, the people shouted to the Executioner, "Lay it on, lay it on, Officer, he cannot feel it; he's a leper!" Excited by the cries of the people, the Executioner worked so with the lash that he died a little later, as much from the last beating as from opening the wounds made at the three different times, which was no great loss to the country.

Examination of Malingerer   (MIII,50)

Not long ago a big scoundrel feigned being deaf, mute and lame. Sometimes by means of a silver instrument he said had come from Barbary (although stamped with the mark of Paris), he spoke so no one could understand him. He was recognized as an imposter and was put in St. Benoist prison and at the request of the Bailiff for the Poor, I went to the prison and examined him with witnesses. We made the following report to the Bureau of the Poor of Paris:

"We, Ambroisé Paré, Counciller and Premier Surgeon of the King, Pierre Pigray, Surgeon-in-Ordinary of his Majesty and Claude Viard, Surgeon of Paris, certify that today, by request of the Procurer of the Poor, have seen and visited in the Prison of St. Benoist, a certain one who would not give his name, aged about forty years, who was found to have a third of right ear cropped. Also a mark on the right shoulder, which we considered made by a hot iron. Moreover he feigned a great trembling of the leg; he claiming it resulting from loss of the thigh bone, which is false, since the bone is complete; and there appearing no evidence that the said trembling came from any previous disease, but is a voluntary motion. Item: we also examined his mouth (since he wished to persuade us his tongue had been pulled out by the roots, which imposture cannot be feigned), but we have found the tongue complete, without any lesion of it, nor of parts serving its motion; always when he wishes to speak, he uses a silver instrument which cannot serve any purpose, except to hinder his address.

Item: said to be deaf, which he is not, since, when we asked him how his ear had been cut, he responded by signs that someone had bitten it off."

After the Authorities of the Bureau received this report by a porter, they had the venerable imposter taken to the hospital of St. Germain-des-Prés and took away his silver instrument. That night he went over the rather high wall and went to Rouen, where he wanted to practice his imposture. He was apprehended, lashed and banished from the Duchy of Normandie, under pain of the noose.

Malingerer Pretending Prolapsed Bowel
(MIII,50)

M. Flecelle,[112] a wise and experienced Doctor of the Faculty of Medicine, asked me one day to go with him to

---

[112] Graduated at Paris 1528; Physician-in-Ordinary (according to his epitaph), to Kings François I, Henri II, François II and Charles IX. At his own request he was a member of the Commission of the Faculty in its quarrel with Paré in 1559. He died March 30, 1562 (Le Paulmier).

the village of Champigny, two leagues from Paris, where
he had a little house. As soon as we arrived and were walking in the court, a big, robust trollop came up asking alms
in honor of St. Fiacre. She lifted her coat and skirt, showing
a great bowel six or more inches long hanging down. This
gave off a liquid like pus of an abscess, which had stained
and fouled her thighs as well as her chemise, so it was most
foul and indecent to see. He asked her how long she had
suffered this illness and she replied, about four years. Then
M. Flecelle contemplating her face and the condition of her
body, being so fleshy and plump-buttocked, knew it was
impossible to put out so much excrement without making
her emaciated, dehydrated and hectic.

Then with a great leap he threw himself angrily on this
strumpet, kicking her several times under the belly, making
the bowel come loose and fall to the ground with sound
and noise and other things. She confessed then that it was
a beef bowel tied in two places. The bowel was filled with a
mixture of blood and milk and punctured in several places
to let the mixture ooze out. He then kicked her several
more times under the bottom and she pretended to be dead.
We went in the house to call some of the people, pretending
to call the police to take her prisoner. Seeing the gate of
the court open, she jumped up as if she had never been
beaten, took off running and was never seen again in
Champigny.

Malinger—Snake in Belly   (MIII,52)

In 1561 a fat-buttocked, fleshy and well developed
strumpet came to this city from Normandy. Going to the
good houses she begged alms of women and ladies, saying
she had a snake in her belly that had got in while she slept
in hemp field. She made them put their hands on her belly

to feel the snake's movements, which writhed and tormented her day and night, as she said. So everyone gave her alms from compassion, proving her skillful deceit. But one honorable and charitable lady took her into her house and called me with M. Houllier, Regent Physician in the Faculty of Medicine and Germain Cheval, Sworn-Surgeon in Paris, to find out if we could chase this dragon out of the body of this poor woman. Having seen her, Dr. Houllier ordered a medicine (that made her have many stools) which finally would make this beast come out, but it did not. The consultants reassembling, concluded I should put a speculum in the vagina. She was put on a table, where her ensign was displayed to introduce the speculum, with which I made a good and ample dilatation, to see if I could perceive head or tail of this beast. Nothing was found, except a voluntary movement which this trollop made with her epigastric muscles. Recognizing the imposture, we retired and agreed this motion could not come from any beast, but was made by her own muscles. To prove the fact more amply, we told her we would give her a much stronger medicine, with the result that she confessed the truth. She was afraid to take stronger medicine, being assured she no longer had the snake. That very evening she left without saying goodbye to her lady, not forgetting to pack her clothes and some of the lady's and thus was the imposture discovered.

Six days later I saw her at the Gate of Montmartre on a pack horse, a leg here, a leg there, her bosom unfurled, going with the fish mongers, I believe, to make her dragon fly, and to return to her country.

Performance of a Magician   (MIII,61)

Not long ago, in the presence King Charles IX and Messrs. le Mareschal de Montmorency, de Rets, the Seigneur de Lausac, M. de Mazille, King's Premier Physician and M. de St. Pris, King's Valet-de-Chambre, I saw things done by an imposter and enchanter that are impossible for men to do without the help of the Devil. These deceived our sight and made false and fantastic things appear to us. The imposter freely confessed to the King that he did these things with the assistance of a spirit to whom he was bound for three more years and who greatly tormented him. He promised the King that when his time was served, he would be a good man. God will forgive him, for it is written, "Thou shall not suffer a witch to live." King Saul was cruelly punished for having talked to the witch. Moses similarly commanded the Hebrews to take pains to exterminate enchanters.

Hemorrhage Arrested Verbally   (MIII,65)

I have seen a man who could stop bleeding from any part of the body by saying words unknown to me.

"Gout" of Lady's Hip   (MIII,211)

When the King (Charles IX—Ed.) was at Bordeaux[113] (1565), I was called with Messrs. Chapelain, Counsellor and Premier Physician of the King, Castellan, Counsellor

---

[113] Bordeaux, now a city of around 260,000 people on the bank of the Garonne, has been the headquarters for famous wines for centuries. Paré visited the city with the Court in 1565 on the way back to Paris on the famous tour with Catherine de' Médicis and young King Charles IX.

and Physician of the King and Premier of the Queen, M. de la Taste, Physician of Bordeaux and M. Nicole Lambert, King's Surgeon-in-Ordinary to examine and advise a lady of about forty years. She was ill with a tumor the size of a pea located outside and below the left hip joint. The tumor and surrounding parts at intervals felt extreme pain as I will describe later. They used every means of appeasing it, calling many Physicians and Surgeons as well as wizards and witches; none could give her relief of her pain. But having heard all this history, I wanted to know what complications followed the peak of the pain, so I took myself to the home of the Lady, accompanied by M. de le Taste. Soon after we arrived her pain took her. She began to scream, to throw herself here and there, making incredible movements. She put her head between her legs and her feet on her shoulders, with many other marvelous movements. This crisis lasted nearly a quarter of an hour during which I tried to determine if swelling or inflammation developed at the site of the pain, but I could ascertain neither, either to sight or touch. It was true that when I touched it, she cried louder. The crisis passed; she remained in a great heat and universal sweat, with lassitude of all her extremities, nor could she move. After seeing such a thing, I remained greatly marveling, as was also the said de la Taste. I asked him what he thought and he replied that he believed a demon tortured this poor creature. This I could not contradict at the time, having never seen nor heard of such a situation. For if this was an epileptic attack it should follow loss of all the senses, with convulsion but this Lady cerebrated well and spoke even better. After having reported this spectacle to Messrs. Chapelain and Castellan, they were greatly astonished. We concluded (seeing that they had tried by several means, which in no wise drew out the pain) that the potential cautery should be applied to this tumor. When I applied it and the crust fell off, a very dark, virulent material drained and she never had another pain.

"Gout"—Pain in Arm   (MIII,212)

A similar thing happened to the wife of the Queen's Coachman at Amboise. On certain days she had pains in her right arm similar to those of the said Lady. She came to Orléans to see Messrs. Chapelain, Castellan and me, begging us to relieve her of the pain, which was so vehement that she wanted to throw herself from the windows, for this reason having a guard with her. We concluded that the potential cautery should be applied to this part, as we had done to the said Lady. I did this, and the opening made, her pain ceased and has since been gone.

Treatment of Shoulder Pain by Vomiting (MIII,225)

I happened to have treated in this city a Gentleman of Geneva who had a severe pain in the left shoulder joint, with weakness of the arm. He had been treated by many Physicians and Surgeons both at Lyon and in this City. He told me that to relieve his pain he had been purged, bled, dieted, treated him with guiac as well as with squill and they had made many applications on the site of the pain. Notwithstanding all the things he had done, they gave him little help. On this I asked him if he had syphilis, since his pain was worse by night than by day, since the cause was a pituitous and cold nature; he replied no. After hearing all the remedies that had been used by learned people I knew no other to order except vomiting. He told me it was difficult to vomit; I advised him to drink heavily and eat many diverse foods at supper, with onions, leeks and such. Then he should drink more of several wines, both sweet and sour, since a great quantity of diversity of food and drink is a cause of vomiting. Some are burning, one decays before the other and the great quantity does not let them be digested in the stomach, so it follows that one vomits more easily. I also advised him to lie down soon after, and that at his first arising he provoke himself to vomit, putting a feather or his finger in his throat. The result would be to throw out with the food great viscid and serous phlegm. He was told to make this debauchment for two or three successive days, for, as Hippocrates said, the second and the next day can eliminate what remained from the first. I told him to continue the emesis once or twice a month and that at times he take in his mouth and chew some yellow mastic, thus to evacuate and diverge the humor which, he said, he felt flow from his head over his shoulder. Also, he should massage his neck and shoulder with brandy in which was infused rosemary, lavender and powdered cloves. Also, he mildly exercise the arm.

Some time later I saw him. He said he had done what I advised and had never found a better way of easing his pain and lost it. Thus all was healed and he used the arm better than ever.

Smallpox, Abscesses of Sternum and Shoulder (MIII,258)

To give you a notable example, I will describe this one, which is one of the most marvelous I have ever seen. The little four or five year old daughter of Claude Piqué, King's Librarian living in the rue St. Jacques in Paris, had been ill with smallpox for about a month. Nature not being able to master the poison, she developed abscesses of the sternum and the shoulder joints where the virulent matter tore and separated all the bones of the sternum and the epiphyses of said bone, with a good portion of the head of the scapula. I did not see this alone, but with M. Miron,[114] at present Counsellor and Premier Physician of the King, Regent Physician of the Faculty of Medicine of Paris (in 1575—Ed.) and Jean Doreau, Surgeon of M. le Comte de Bryane. In their presence I saw and autopsied this girl, in whom I found what I described above.

Smallpox, Osteomyelitis and Fractures
(MIII,258)

Roland Marie, Merchant Spectacle-maker, dwelling near the Palais,[115] took me to his daughter, aged four years and two months. Her whole body was covered with pustules and smallpox. The bones of the arms and legs were ab-

---

[114] Marc Miron, son of François Miron, Premier-Physician of Charles VII. Marc was born at Tours and got his degree in 1558. He went to Poland with the duc d'Anjou (later Henri III) where the duc became King of Poland. When Henri III became King of France, he made Miron his Premier-Physician. Miron went to Nancy in 1575 with Paré to treat the King's sister, the Duchess de Lorraine in her last illness. He died on November 1, 1608 (Le Paulmier, 84).

The Latin edition (1582) of Paré's "Complete Works" was dedicated to Miron by Guillemeau (see Doe, 156).

[115] The Palais, formerly the house of the King, occupied the site on the Ile de la Cité now termed the de Justice, although by Paré's time the court had moved out and the Parlement was installed in the old royal residence. More buildings have encroached on the court surrounding St. Louis' 13th century St. Chapelle. Paré lived just across St. Michel's bridge from the Palais, and no doubt had a view of it from his windows.

scessed, putrid and fractured, accompanied by a high fever. I did not want to touch her; the next day she died.

Smallpox; Internal Pustules   (MIII,260)

A while ago I saw two girls aged four and seventeen years, with M. Richard Hubert, Sworn-Surgeon of Paris. After their death we found their interior parts all covered with crusted pustules, resembling those seen outside.

Intestinal Worms   (MIII,264)

But long and thick or flat, sometimes they (worms— ED.) fill the whole length of the intestines and such are like a mucous and glairy substance. Truly I saw one that came out of a woman, that resembled a serpent more than six feet long. This is not surprising, since the ancients wrote of having seen them as long as the intestines, which is normally seven times the length of the body. I know this from having seen it and shown it in public anatomic dissections at the Schools of Medicine of this City.

Lepers—Strange Heat of   (MIII,280)

Some have strange heat of the body, as I witnessed by sight. One of these kept a fresh apple in his house for an hour, after which it was dried out and wrinkled as if it had been in the sun for eight hours.

Laxatives Acting on Baby Through Milk   (MIII,288)

Similarly one sees, when Doctors want to purge an infant still at the breast, giving laxative medicines to the nurse makes their milk medicinal and laxative. I recently saw a sick nurse for whom the Doctors ordered laxative medicines; after nursing the infant had diarrhea that was hard to arrest. This constrained them from treating another nurse until the medicine had ceased acting.

Theriac in Dog-Bite   (MIII,311)

And to prove my point, I offer the history of one of the maids of Mademoiselle deGron, native of this City of Paris, who was bitten by a mad dog in the right leg. The dog set his teeth deeply in the flesh. This was cured without any complication by using theriac.[116] This theriac I used in the detersive and other medications, to the end of her cure.

Snake Bite—Personal History   (MIII,314)

I wish to recite another history here to instruct the young surgeon. King Charles being at Montpellier,[117] I was bitten

---

[116] Theriac was a complicated distilled and fermented drug used as a preventive as well as a curative medication against "venoms." It thus was employed in plague, against bites of animals and indeed, against almost all deadly wounds or ailments. Paré was almost as credulous of its efficacy as he was dubious of other nostrums such as mummy and bezoar. He listed at least three formulas for its preparation (MII, 599, 600 and MIII, 368).

[117] Montpellier, a city of about 100,000 inhabitants on the Mediterranean coast. The site of an ancient Medical School, Montpellier inaugurated granting of degrees in 1220, twenty years earlier than Paris. In the 14th century the School took an intellectual lead over Salerno and Bologna. Guy de Chauliac studied at Bologna and Paris before becoming famous in surgery at Montpellier in the 14th century. Paré's contemporaries, the Royal Physicians Castellan and Chapelain both graduated at Montpellier. Paré himself visited the city in 1564 on the long Court tour with Charles IX and Catherine de' Médicis and left the account of having been bitten by a viper.

by a viper at the end of the index finger between the nail and the flesh, in the house of an Apothecary named Farges. He dispensed theriac and I asked to see the vipers he used in its preparation. He showed me a great number that he kept in a stone vessel. I took one out, wishing to see its teeth, which are in the superior mandible of its jaw, covered by a little membrane in which it holds its venom, which it expresses, as I have said, into the part in which it has just made an opening.

Having received this bite, I suddenly felt an extreme pain as much from the sensibility of the part as from the venom. I tied the finger very tightly above the wound to make it bleed and force out the venom and to prevent it going upward. Then I demanded some old theriac which I dissolved in brandy, held by one of Farges' servants. I soaked some cotton in the mixtures and applied it to the wound. After a few days I was cured without any complication, by this remedy alone.

Bite of an Adder   (MIII,320)

The King being at Moulins,[118] M. le Fèvre, King's Physician-in-Ordinary, M. Jacques le Roy, his Surgeon-in-Ordinary and I were called to treat a cook of Madame de Castelpers. While picking a basket of hops to make a salad, he was bitten on the hand by an adder. He sucked the blood of the wound and soon after his tongue swelled so he could scarcely speak nor be understood. Moreover, the whole arm to the shoulder enlarged and swelled greatly, as does a soufflé. The patient felt extreme pain and fell twice in

---

[118] Moulins, a town about 35 Km. north of Vichy. Paré visited the place with the Court in 1566 when Coligny was tried by the privy Council for the murder of the duc de Guise three years earlier.

our presence from the heart failing, as if dead. His face and whole body had a jaundiced and leaden color.

Seeing these complications, we said death was imminent, nevertheless, he was not left without help. His mouth was washed with theriac in white wine then he was given some to drink in brandy. In his turgid arm I made several deep incisions, even in the bite and let the blood (which was only serous) flow freely. These were washed with brandy in which theriac and methridat were dissolved. The patient was put into a well-warmed bed to sweat and was kept awake to prevent the venom from going with the natural heat to the heart. And truly, the next day the complications cleared and the incisions healed soon afterward.

Facial Blemish (Acne?) Treated with Cantharides   (MIII,328)

Some years ago a damoiselle came to Paris with her face broken out with great sapphires or pustules, with such redness that many who saw her thought her to have leprosy. They even forbade her to enter the Church of the parish. She called M. Jacque Houllier and Robert Greaume, Regent Physician in the Faculty of Medicine, with Étienne de la Rivière and Germain Cheval, Sworn Paris Surgeons, to give aid in her illness. She showed us many recipes for remedies she had taken trying to be cured. We examined her thoroughly and concluded that she had no leprosy. To treat her eruption one should apply a vesicatory made of cantharides to her whole face to draw out the matter from the pustules as well as the superfluous humors that also imbued all her face. This was done.

Three or four hours after the vesicatory had taken effect she had an amazing burning in the bladder and great swelling of the neck of the uterus, with severe spasms. She vomited, voided and purged incessantly, threw herself about as if she had been afire and was irrational and feverish. I was amazed at the effect and called back the Medical and Surgical Consultants. Seeing that these complications resulted from cantharides applied for its vesicatory effect, I was advised to give her a great deal of milk to drink as well as by clyster and by injection into the bladder and the vagina. Also she was bathed in moderately hot water in which had been boiled linseed, roots and leaves of mallows and marshmallows, Mars violets, henbane, purbane and lettuce. She remained in it a long time, causing her pain to stop. Then she was put in bed and dried and rose ointment and poplar salve containing oxycrate applied to her loins and genital areas to reduce the intemperance of these parts. By these means the other complications cleared.

Her face was entirely blistered and drained a great amount of purulent matter. By this means she lost the great facial disfigurement she had suffered. After she was healed we gave her certifications that she had never been attacked by leprosy. She soon returned to her home, was married, has since had two fine infants and lives still without showing any sign of having had her face flayed.

Bite of Vive (a Sea Fish)   (MIII,331)

Recently the wife of M. Fromaget, Registrar of Requests of the Palais, was wounded by a viver (a sea fish— ED.) on her ring finger. It quickly swelled greatly, with great flushing and little pain. Seeing the swelling extend to the hand she feared such an accident that recently befell an old neighbor, and sent for me. The widow of the late M. Bargelonne, Lieutenant Particular of the Châtelet of

Paris had been similarly stung. Because of negligence she had developed gangrene and mortification of the whole arm and died miserably. Having reached Mme. Fromaget and learned the cause of her trouble, I promptly applied to the finger and hand a poultice of a large onion roasted under the coals and mixed with a little theriac. The next morning I had her soak her hand in hot water to draw out the venom. Afterward I made several superficial incisions around the finger. Then I applied leeches to the incisions, and they drew out sufficient blood. I applied theriac dissolved in brandy; the next day I found her finger and arm deflated and free of pain. Some days later she was entirely healed.

I also similarly treated the cook of M. de Soussy, Treasurer of l'Espargue, who also was stung by a vive. His whole arm was swollen and inflamed to the shoulder, and in a few days he also was cured.

Test of Bezoar of Charles IX   (MIII,341)

The late King being in his town of Clermont[119] in Auvergne, a Gentleman brought him a Bezoar stone from Spain. He said it was good against all poisons and esteemed it greatly. Being in the King's room, he called me and asked me if he could find some certain and simple drug against all poisons. I answered, no; saying that there are many sorts and kinds of venoms, one must oppose some of them in one way, others in another. I told him that poisons do not produce the same effect nor produce these effects in a similar way. Some operate by an excess of elementary

[119] Clermont, presently designated Clermont-Ferrand, a city of 114,000 inhabitants in Auvergne, 380 Km. south of Paris. The described incident probably occurred during the young King Charles' tour of the country in 1564-1565.

qualities of which they are composed; others operate by their own specific qualities, occult and secret, following no rule, and according to their diversity acted contrarily. If they were hot they were cured by cold remedies and the cold by hot remedies, and thus as to other qualities.

The Lord who had the stone wished despite my reasons to prove it was specific against all poisons. So I told the King that he could try it on some criminal who was going to be hanged. He promptly sent for M. de la Trousse, Provost of his house and asked him if he had someone who deserved the noose. He told him he had in his prison a cook who had stolen two silver dishes from the house of his Master, whose domestic he was, and who was to be hanged and strangled the next day.

The King told him he wished to experiment with a stone said to be an antidote against all poisons and that he would know of the condemned cook if he wished to take some certain poison and immediately afterward, an antidote. If he escaped, he would have his life saved. The cook agreed willingly, saying he would like much better to die in prison of poison than to be strangled in the sight of people.

An apothecary then gave him a potion of a certain poison and immediately some of the Bezoar stone. Having these two drugs in his stomach, he began to vomit and then moved his bowels with great cramps, saying his body was on fire, demanding water to drink, which was not refused him. An hour after being told the cook had taken this drug, I asked M. de la Trousse to let me go see him, which he permitted, accompanied by three of his archers. I found the poor cook moving like a beast on all fours, his tongue out of his mouth, his eyes and face flaming, trying constantly to vomit, bathed in cold sweat, pouring blood from his ears, nose, mouth, anus and penis. I gave him about a pint of oil to drink, thinking to help him and save his life, but it did him no good, as it was given too late. He died miserably, crying that it was better to die on the gallows. He lived about seven hours.

Being dead, I opened his body in the presence of M. de la Trousse and four of his Archers. I found the bottom of his stomach black, hard and dry as if it had been cauterized, which let me know he had swallowed sublimate, by the complications of which he had lost his life.

Thus as the experience showed, the Spanish stone had no virtue. The King ordered it thrown in the fire, which was done.

Abscesses of Liver and Lungs in Plague
(MIII,361)

When one opens dead bodies (of plague victims—Ed.) one finds in nearly all of them abscesses of the internal parts, such as the liver and lungs, made by putrefaction acquired by the mixing of the blood and principally by the ambient air corrupted and altered, and not by cannon powder nor bullets, which some consider poisoned.

(First description of liver and lung abscesses in plague— Malgaigne.)

Odor of Plague Victim, Paré's Syncope
(MIII,380)

I will describe here, as an example of danger one runs in visiting the infected, what happened to me once going to see a plague victim. He had a pestiferous bubo in the right groin and two large carbuncles of the abdomen. On arriving, I lifted the sheet and the coverlet and was struck by a terrible fetid odor, produced as much by the sweat of his body as by the putrid exhalation of the pus of both the abscess and the carbuncles. Being enveloped by this vapor, I fell to the ground as if dead, as do those who faint, that is to say, whose heart fails, but without any pain, nor cardiac change, a manifest sign that only the animal spirit was offended. After I got up it seemed that the house turned from top to bottom and I had to hold to one of the posts of the patient's bed, or I would have fallen again. Having regained my spirits in a little while, I sneezed ten or twelve times so hard my nose bled. This was why, in my opinion, the pestilential vapor did not affect me. But I leave to the reader if death was not averted because of the strength of the expulsive force of my brain, since all my senses, and especially the animal spirits which are the instruments of life, failed me for a moment.

Sudden Death in Plague   (MIII,388)

By the violence of this sudden and prompt venom, those who are struck sometimes die unexpectedly; even while eating, drinking and discharging their duties, they fall dead walking the streets and temples. I saw this recently when the King (Charles IX—Ed.) was at Lyon.[120]

Sometimes also, the complications clear and it seems that the patient is doing well and of good cheer. This happened to one of the Queen's damoiselles, named la Mare, when

---

[120] Lyon—Paré was in this strategic city at least twice, in 1542 on his way to Perpignan and again in 1565 on the two year tour with the court to show the child-king Charles IX to the country. They found the city in an attack by the plague.

the King was at the Castle of Roussillon. She was struck by the plague, having a bubo in the groin, which quieted down. On the third day she said she felt well except for a little difficulty voiding, (due to the inflammation of the urinary tract). She walked about her room mentally clear. Nevertheless that same day she gave up her spirit to God, which was the reason we promptly left that place. (see also pg. 140—ED.)

Plague, Bleeding and Purging   (MIII,411)

I would like to tell you of what I observed on the trip to Bayonne,[121] which I made with my King (Charles IX —ED.) in 1565. I inquired of Physicians, Surgeons and Barbers of all the towns we passed where the plague had been, if they were advised to bleed the pestilent. They told me that nearly all those who were bled or severely purged were dead and those who were not bled nor purged nearly all recovered. This made it appear that the plague came from an evil of the air, and not of corruption of the humors.

---

[121] Bayonne, 8 Km. inland from the now famous costal resort of Biarritz in the southwest corner of France, was the focus of the Court tour of France in 1564-1565. After wintering in Montpellier, the vast entourage reached Bayonne on April 9, 1565. Late in May Catherine de' Médicis' daughter Elizabeth, Queen of Spain, arrived accompanied by the duc d'Alva and a Spanish delegation. On June 3rd the formal conference occurred, the Spanish pressing Catherine to undertake total Huguenot extermination. It was suspected that decisions made here led to the 1572 St. Bartholomew's Day Massacre, but Alva reported to Philippe that he failed to get Catherine's agreement to any repression and found her "more than cold" toward the Holy Religion.

During the visit Paré toured the area, going among other places to Biarritz to treat the Prince de la Roche-sur-Yon. Here he observed whaling, later described in his book on *Monsters and Prodigies*, and sent a whale vertebra home for his museum.

Plague, Treatment with Anchovy Brine
(MIII,415)

Moreover, the said Eroüard (Gilbert Eroüard, Physician of Montpellier) told me he had used this recipe (of anchovy brine—Ed.) in many cases. I even gave some to two children of M. de la Terrasse, King's Master of Requests, who had the plague and they were cured.

Plague, Effect of Nosebleed   (MIII,419)

Sometimes the blood escapes spontaneously (from the nose—Ed.) since it is hot, subtile and bilious when Nature makes a crisis. I saw this happen to M. de Fontaine, Chevalier of the Order of the King (his Majesty being at Bayonne). He had a continous pestilential fever accompanied by several carbuncles over his body, and for two days bled constantly from the nose. With this flux his fever ended with a profuse sweat. Soon afterward the carbuncles suppurated. I dressed him and by the grace of God, he recovered. (See also pg. 191)

Dysentery, Origin of Intestinal Hemorrhage
(MIII,422)

That which I have seen many times happened especially at the camp at Amiens (1558—Ed.) where many died of diarrhea. This was very contagious and especially to those who went to the privies after those who passed such excrement. Wishing to know the source of such large quantities of blood, I opened some after death and found the mouths of the mesenteric arteries and veins open and swollen where they joined the intestines, in the form of little cotyledons the size of small peas. When I squeezed them blood squirted out, and thus I saw the route by which blood was evacuated in the stools. M. le Grand, King's Surgeon-in-Ordinary, who was with me at the camp at the command of the late King Henry (II—ED.) saved many. Among other remedies, he made them drink milk of shod cattle. He often had this injected into the rectum to neutralize the acidity of the humor. (See also pg. 141—ED.)

Large Plague Carbuncles: Personal Case (MIII,436)

I have seen carbuncles whose scars occupied nearly half of the back, others drawing the clavicles toward the breast and having so deeply eroded the subjacent tissues that one could see the uncovered trachea. Others occupied half of the epigastric muscles and the falling crust revealing the exposed peritoneum. I myself had a carbuncle (which a marginal note attributed to the plague—ED.) on my belly, the persisting scar being as large as the palm of a hand. When they are so great and enormous, they most often are fatal.

Plague, Deep Tissue Necrosis (MIII,437)

At the Hôtel-Dieu in Paris I saw plague victims who appeared to have tumors of the excretory organs, who the next day showed nothing. When the patients did I was curious to search the part for the cause to death. Truly, having made a sufficiently deep incision, in some I found the flesh to be burned as if an actual cautery had passed over it.

Plague, Mode of Death   (MIII,438)

If the brain is attacked, frenzy and madness follow, then death. If the venom attacks the urinary tract, the victim dies of suppression of urine. This happened at Roussillon Castle (outside Lyon—ED.) to one of the Queen's damoiselles of whom I spoke earlier (See pg. 136—ED.).

Plague, Stomach Lesion and Purpura (MIII,438)

Also if the carbuncle ruptures into the stomach, that is mortal. This happened to the Governor of Dames (Nursing Sisters—ED.) of the Hôtel Dieu of Paris when I was there treating the patients. Here was a tall, straight, strong and powerful young monk of the Order of St. Victor who developed a continuous fever. His tongue became black, dry, scaly and rough from the extreme heat of his fever and the putrid vapor ascending from the internal parts to the mouth (for as the vulgar say, when a furnace is hot enough the mouth resents it). His tongue protruded like a dog that has run far, and was very altered. He was perpetually thirsty, with great weakening of the heart and constant vomiting. He died on the third day in generalized convulsion of all extremities.

Seeing the poor monk die so rapidly and considering his complications so cruel, the Dames suspected he had been poisoned. Being informed of this, the Governors of Hôtel-Dieu ordered the Monk's body to be opened, to know the truth. They called a Physician and a Surgeon to do this with me. Having opened it, we found at the bottom of the stomach an area like that left by a potential cautery, with a scar or crust as large as a fingernail and the rest of the stomach strongly contracted and hard. Then all concluded that he had been poisoned with sublimate or arsenic, since the scar penetrated very deeply. As I was sewing up the body I noticed many little black spots scattered over his body. When I recalled the consultants to observe these spots, they said and affirmed that this was purpura. But the Physician and Surgeon told me they were bites of fleas or bed-bugs, to which I could not agree because he had so many of them. To prove my point I took a needle, pushed it deeply into the skin in several places and lifting it up, cut with scissors and found the flesh beneath to be very black. Also we considered the lividity of the nose, ears, the nails and even the whole body being darker than usual at death from other causes. His face changed so it was almost impossible to recognize him. Now they changed the opinion and reported that the Monk had died of a plague carbuncle and not of any poison.

Dysentery, Source of Intestinal Bleeding (MIII,449)

When I was at the camp at Amiens this (dysentery —ED.) attacked many strong and powerful soldiers. I dissected some of them after death to find the source of such a quantity of blood that could escape. I found the mouths of the mesenteric veins and arteries opened and elevated, or tumefied where they reached the intestines into little cotyledons, which when compressed yielded pure blood. (See also pg. 138—ED.)

Plague, Murder and Robbery (MIII,458)

Those who would like recent examples can get them from the inhabitants of Lyon on the trip the King made (1564 —ED.). Also in this city of Paris are found people who with the aid of such masters, made it understood that someone who was an enemy had the plague, without being ill in any way. On the day he had to come to court or to do something requiring his presence, he was taken up and carried by force to the Hôtel-Dieu by these gallants, against such resistance as he could make, being one against many. And if by chance he implored the aid and sympathy of witnesses, the thieves and murderers prevented it and shouted louder then he, so he was not understood. They were given to understand that the illness had made him mad and maniacal, to make them run away; thus they could take him to the Hôtel-Dieu and put him to bed with the plague victims. He died some days later, as much from despair as from the infected air, having been sold and bought before his death for the cash he carried.

Plague, Maddened Patient Killing
(MIII,460)

Along this line, I have learned that not long since, a Priest of St. Eustace's parish in this city was sick of plague in the Hôtel-Dieu. Becoming maniacal he got out of bed and taking a dagger, struck many poor patients in their beds, killing three. Had he not been seen and overpowered by a surgeon of the hospital (who in seizing him was stabbed in the abdomen, of which he thought he would die) he would have slain more. But as soon as he was taken and his fury lessened, he gave up his spirit.

Plague, Suicide During Frenzy   (MIII,460)

Another case no less horrible happened on rue Merciere at Lyon, where Amy Basten, wife of a Surgeon who had died of the plague, was taken with the same contagion six days later. She fell into a dreamy state, then into frenzy and went to the window of her room, holding and tormenting her baby in her arms. Her neighbors who saw her begged her not to hurt him, but instead of taking their advice, she hurled him heedlessly to the ground and then leaped after him. Thus the mother and the infant died.

Introduction to Discourse on Mummy and Unicorn (MIII,468)

Monsieur, (M. Christophe des Ursins[122]—Ed.) you remember that on the last day of August 1580, between the Abbey of Chally (Chaalis) and Armenonville (Ermenonville, 44 Km. from Paris—Ed.), one of your huge horses reared and toppled upon you and you fell on rough, sharp gravel on the small of the back. The horse being good and spirited, began to get up, but no sooner raised than he half fell again and gave you a second injury. Except for the prompt and faithful assistance of one of your Gentlemen named de Selles, who promptly dismounted and with great effort pulled you out from beneath, your person would have been in great danger. Immediately on falling you were in a faint, with failure of heart and speech. You were carried to your house where you were put to bed, the same complications recurring and persisting for four hours. During this time, thanks to the diligence of your companion

---

[122] Christophe Jouvenel des Ursins, Seigneur de la Chapelle-Gautier, of Doüe and of Armenonville, Marquis de Traisnel, Governor of Paris and Lieutenant-General of the Ile de France. Oldest son of François Jouvenel des Ursins. He participated in the defense of Metz, 1552, married Madelaine de Luxembourg in 1557. He died in 1588 (Le Paulmier, p. 105—Packard, p. 197).

(certainly a Lady of great virtue) nothing imaginable was omitted to help you. For this Doctors and Surgeons were called from nearby such as Senlis and Dampmartin and Madame la Connestable even sent you M. le Fèvre, King's Surgeon-in-Ordinary, who was then at Chantilly. He bled you and used other remedies proper for such injuries. Nothing was neglected to sedate the pains and resolve the bruised blood spreading through the loins, and even into the lower belly and thighs. Seeing that you did not feel this and rally as quickly as desired, they sent for me in Paris.

Having received your letters, for the service I owed you and all your house, I promptly mounted horse. On arriving I found a great tumefaction and doughy swelling a little above the sacrum. I was of the opinion to open it to let out a great deal of clotted blood and serum which, if remaining under the skin, can cause putrefaction, gangrene and other such mortal complications which can develop in such great contusions. The opening made, over the space of ten or twelve days no less than a pint of blood clot and serum drained each time you were dressed. The napkins and kerchiefs folded four or five times were soaked as if they had been taken from a pail of water. Considering this, I began to fear that your whole body might melt, thus leaving you tabetic. Realizing also that this material drained from many great cavities, it was necessary to make other incisions. This was explained to the said Lady and your son-in-law, M. de Paleseau and Madame your daughter, who were very anxious over your health. I asked them, as much in respect for the apparent danger as for your importance, which is one of the greatest in France, that we get more advice. At which the said Lady, wishing to spare nothing, immediately wrote the King that if it pleased his Majesty, he should send M. Pigray, a man very wise in Surgery. This the King did willingly. Also he sent M. de Mouron, a man esteemed among those wise and well informed in Medicine and Surgery and also M. Hautin, Regent Physician in the Faculty of Medicine, Messrs. Cointeret and le Fort,[123] Surgeons. They came and after seeing, examining and studying your injury, concurred unanimously with us that it was more than necessary to make new openings. This would make it easier to wash out the cavities under the abraded and contused skin. God favored our labors and thus you were healed, thanks to God.

When beginning to get about well, your pains diminishing, you honored me by discussing may good things. Among others you asked why they had not given you Mummy to drink at the time of your fall. Then I replied that I was glad of it, since it could do much more harm than good, since it is the flesh of purulent and cadaverous dead bodies, —etc.

Sword Wound of Orbit   (MIII,488)

On March 12, 1582, M. Bernault de l'Estelle, a Gentleman of the Company of M. le Maréschal de Biron, fencing at the Maréschal's place, got a contused wound in the left eye penetrating to near the surface of the fourth cervical vertebra. This was made by the Baron du Bouluet of Quercy with a guarded epée at the tip of which was a round, flat button a good inch wide. Moreover the blow did not pass nor break through the skin completely, but left a little livid, black tumor the size of a filbert. Also, the entire head and neck swelled and could not turn, from the blood that spread

---

[123] Rodolphe le Fort of Senlis became a Paris Surgeon and finally Provost of the College of Surgeons. He died June 22, 1606.

between the muscles of the neck. The Lord bled by nose and mouth and was greatly stunned by the blow. As soon as the Lord Baron, a strong and powerful man, had struck he wished to withdraw the epée but could do so only with great difficulty after two separate attempts, because the bones of the orbit were broken and pushed back by the great violence of the blow.

My Lord the Maréschal sent for me to come to his house to treat the wounded man. Having arrived, he asked me to take as much care as if he were one of his own children. Then I promised him I would be as solicitous as if it were himself. Having examined him I concluded, with M. Paradis, Surgeon of My Lord the Maréschal and Solin Crinel, Surgeon of French troops (men greatly experienced in Surgery, from their long experiences, who worked with me until the cure was complete) that he should be bled from the cephalic vein on the side of the injury. Pigeon blood (which is a true eye balm) was put in the eye and on the neighboring parts, egg white beaten in rose-water and plantain. The whole head was treated with a liniment of oxyrrhodinum. After cutting his hair a plaster of diachalcitoes dissolved in rose oil and vinegar was applied to prevent inflammation of the interior parts of the brain. We also made an opening at the spot where the epée had failed to come out, from which drained a good quantity of black, curdled blood. This was held open until we could see the head and neck deflate. The complications passing, we did several other things I will omit for brevity.

I will not pass on without saying that Messrs. Pigray, Cointeret, Le Fort, Dioniau, Viard, Nicholas Marc and several other Physicians and Surgeons came to see this wound treated, without loss of sight, which is truly a remarkable thing. He was cured, thanks to God, in twenty-four days, and that without any part of the bone coming out, which is still more remarkable. If someone should ask me how it happened, I would reply that perhaps the orbital bones which had been displaced could also have been replaced as the epée was withdrawn.

Child Crushed by Coach Wheel   (MIII,489)

On June 7, 1582, the twenty-six month old son of Mathurin le Beau, Merchant Milliner living at the Sign of the Silver Crown in rue St. Denis, was in the middle of the street when the wheels of a coach loaded with five Gentlemen passed across his body. The people cried to the Coachman, who stopped his horses, pulled them back and the wheel again went over the baby's body. He was carried into his father's house, thought to be dead and eviscerated. I was called immediately to treat the child. When I examined him very carefully I could find no fracture nor dislocation anywhere in his body. I immediately sent to the Paris gate to get a sheep. I had it skinned, and after rubbing the infant's body with oil of rose and of myrtle, I wrapped him naked in the hot sheep skin. Then I gave him oxycrate to drink instead of Mummy to prevent the blood from curdling and congealing in the body. In addition, I told the mother to keep him from sleeping as much as possible for at least four or five hours, so the blood would not run so much to the interior of the body (which she did). Moreover, I applied fomentations of resolving herbs and plasters proper for contusions, to dissolve the bruised blood.

Three or four days later seeing that the child could not hold himself up, and still less walk, I called M. Piètre, Regent Physician in the Faculty of Medicine, a man of excellent knowledge, who ordered some little medication for him, for he was very constipated. We feared the retention of excrements resulted from a lesion of the spine and nerves which loosen and expel excrements. Patients who have broken or dislocated their vertebrae often let their excrements go involuntarily, at other times they are retained without power to evacuate them. I have seen this several times. I have also seen that from great contusion the ribs can separate from the vertebrae, where they are joined. So the failure to support himself and walk made me fear I had not found the evil by sight and touch. Knowing that two eyes see more than one, I called Jean Cointeret and Jacques Guillemeau, King's Surgeons, as well experienced in Surgery as they have in Paris. They came and examined the child, on whom they found no fracture or dislocation. Thus the treatment was pursued to the end and he was healed, thanks to God. He walked as he did before he was hurt.

Unicorns Horn—Test of Effect against Poisons   (MIII,505)

In supposing that there is a variety of horns of unicorns, and that everyone could have some, it remains to know if they have such virtues and efficacies against venoms and poisons as are attributed to them. I say they do not. This I will prove by experience, authority and reason.

To begin with experience, I can certify after having proved it many times, never to have found any effect in the horn supposedly of the unicorn. Many hold that if one soaked it in water and with this water make a circle on a table, one then put in this circle a scorpion, spider or a toad, the beast would die, and that they will not pass over the circle, and even that the toad would burst. I have experimented and found this to be false and untrue, for these animals will pass and repass out of the circuit of the circle and not die. Moreover, not contenting myself with putting a toad in the circuit of water in which the unicorn had been soaked, over which he passed and repassed, I put him to soak in a vessel full of water where the horn of the unicorn had soaked and left him in the water for three days, at the end of which the toad was as gay as when I put him there.

Some told me that possibly the horn was not of a true unicorn. To which I reply that that of St. Denis[124] in France, that of the King, held in great repute and those of Parisian merchants, which they sell at great prices, are not true horns of unicorns, for it is those I have tested. And if one does not want to believe me, let him try it as I did and know the truth against the lie.

Unicorns' Horn, Supposed Cure of Eczema (MIII,506)

To prove my point, there is an honest woman merchant of unicorns' horns in this city, living on the bridge of

---

[124] St. Denis, a suburb 11 Km. north of Paris to which St. Denis, the first bishop of Lutece (Roman name for Paris) walked with his head in his hands after having been beheaded at Montmartre. An abbey was founded there in the 7th century and the basilica became the mortuary of French Kings. Their tombs became very elaborate, that of Catherine de' Médicis and Henri II being especially noteworthy. The tombs were desecrated during the Revolution, but the most precious were saved and hidden, to be restored later by Louis 18th.

In November, 1567, the Huguenots under Condé and Coligny marched on Paris and camped at St. Denis. There on November 10th they were attacked by a much larger army of Catholics, but the seventy-five year old Constable Montmorency planned badly and was himself mortally wounded by a pistol ball that fractured his spine, paralyzing him. Paré treated him through his last few days.

Change,[125] who has a great number of small and large ones. She always carries a large piece attached to a silver chain which usually soaks in a pitcher full of water, of which she gives willingly enough to all who ask it. Recently a poor woman asked for some unicorn water. It happened that she had given it all away but did not want to put off this poor woman who with clasped hands begged it of her to give to stop the eczema that covered the whole face of her own little infant. In place of the unicorn water, she gave her river water in which she had not soaked the unicorn's horn. Nevertheless, this river water did not fail to cure the baby's illness, for ten or twelve days later the poor woman came to thank Madam the merchant for her unicorn water, telling her that her infant was all healed.

Potential Cautery—Discovery of its Preparation   (MIII,582)

Then I begged him (a chemist—Ed.) affectionately to describe it to me; he replied that he could not, as this was one of the greatest secrets, but he would give me some when I needed it. Then I prayed him give me one, which he did. I applied it to the arm of one of my servants to try it. I declare to God that in no more than half an hour it made an ulcer that would admit the finger down to the bone, and this cautery was no larger than a pea. It left a soft humid scar as the philosopher had told me. When I knew its effect

---

[125] Bridge of Change, a bridge across the north limb of the Seine connecting the Ile de la Cité with the right bank opposite St. Michel's bridge crossing to the left. The original bridge, finished in the 9th century, carried houses on each side of the roadway, and especially silversmiths, who changed money, hence its name. It led into the Châtelet on the right bank.

by experience. I returned immediately to find this master and begged the recipe of him at whatever cost, that he give me the description of this cautery with the manner of making it. He refused me flatly; as much as I showed my desire to have his secret, the more he raised it. Finally I told him I would give him enough velour to make a pair of breeches. For this he granted my wish on condition that I would never tell it to another and that I would not write it in my book, reproaching me that I was too liberal in communicating my knowledge. To this I responded that if our predecessors had done so, we would know few things—etc.

And if someone wishes to object to not having kept my promise to this Chemist, that I tell it to no one nor write of it, I reply that when he sold it, it was mine. And especially I think I did not wrong him; on the contrary he and I have done something that will serve the public.

Near Asphyxia—Charcoal Fire   (MIII,661)

On March 10, 1575, I was called with M. Greaulme, Regent Physician in the Faculty of Medicine to the house of M. du Hamel, Advocate in the Court of Parlement at Paris to examine and make a report of two of their servants, one a clerk and the other a groom whom they estimated to be dead, since they had no sign of pulse. They had a universal coldness of their entire bodies, without speech or any movement. Moreover having lead colored facies, from the fact that on pinching or pulling hair rudely they felt nothing, so that all present estimated them to be dead.

But the dispute was in the manner of death, for the said du Hamel said they had been suffocated; others thought them to have murdered one another; others philosophised their having been taken with apoplexy. I asked if they had not made a fire of charcoal, to which each replied not knowing. The said du Hamel hearing this, went to search their room, (which was very small and closed) where he found under the table a large brazier still containing charcoal not all burned. Seeing this it was the conclusion of all that the cause of this disaster would prove to be nothing else than the malignant fumes of glowing charcoal that had thus dazed and suffocated them.

When one put his hand on the region of the heart, as much by the warmth which persisted there as by the small beating one perceived, he knew these still to be alive and was advised to assist them promptly. To do this they were made by artifice to open their mouths (which were held strongly closed, the teeth locked) into which la hiere and theriac dissolved in rectified brandy was injected with a quill and syringe, to make them swallow it. Then they began to move and to excrete mucous and viscid excrements by mouth and nose. Then they began to bubble as cabbages boil in a pot. They were made to swallow emetics and quantities of oxymel; they were beaten with hand and knee rudely enough on the back toward the last dorsal vertebra and the first of the lumbar near which lies the orifice of the stomach turning toward its posterior part. Finally, by virtue of the emetics as well as contraction of the stomach, they were forced to disgorge. This being done, they spewed up viscid yellow phlegm flecked with blood. Also the tuft of feathers were thrust into the nose and produced euphorbus to stimulate the expulsive force of the brain to discharge itself. By this means they began sneezing, discharging great quantities of matter by the nose. They moreover were aroused with oil of mint, drawn to quintessence, rubbed in their palate, as well as on the breast and into the gullet with a feather greased with some drops of the said oil. In addition they were treated by friction made on the arms, thighs and legs and along the spine of the back, also by acid and strong clysters by which they emptied their bowels copiously. Then they began to speak and to return to themselves, to drink, to eat and become natural little by little. In the execution of all such things we were wonderfully assisted by Jacques Guillemeau, Licensed Surgeon of Paris and M. Jean de St. Germain, Master Apothecary of Paris, a good man and helpful to patients. In the afternoon M. Thibault and M. Hautin, Regent Physician in the Faculty of Medicine (men learned in Medicine as in Surgery) were called to consult with us as to what remained to be done. They approved all we had done, point by point, and agreed with us as to their future care, by cardac restoratives and comforting spirits, etc.—.

Paré Poisoned (MIII,662)

After the capture of Rouen (Oct. 26, 1562) I found myself at dinner in a group including some who hated me to death for the Religion.[126] They gave me cabbage containing sublimate or arsenic. At first bite I noticed nothing; the second, I felt a great heat and burning, a great astriction of

---

[126] For a variety of reasons, particularly this chance remark, a "slip of the pen" as some have termed it, Paré has been called a Huguenot. Contemporaries wished to claim him for one side or the other. Later historians have drawn conclusions variously, as Packard reported (p. 84). Malgaigne considered him Catholic. Parkard cited the report of Le Paulmier (p. 80) who found a note of Paré himself that he considered settled the argument beyond all question on the Huguenot side. Rereading the testimony (Le Paulmier 243) however, leaves one very unwilling to consider it a declaration of faith. Certainly if Paré had thus in 1575 proclaimed himself a Huguenot, he could hardly have continued living under Catholic rites as he did for the next fifteen years.

the mouth and especially the gullet and the stinking taste of the good drug. Having perceived it, I immediately took a glass of water and of wine and washed my mouth and drank a large quantity and promptly went to the house of the nearest apothecary. As soon as I left the plate of cabbage was thrown on the ground. At the Apothecary's shop I vomited and quickly drank about a pint of oil, kept it in my stomach a while and threw it up. The oil prevented the sublimate from adhering to the wall of the stomach. That done, I ate and drank a large amount of milk to which I added butter and two egg yolks. And that is how I escaped the hand of the poisoner, and subsequently I never took cabbage nor any other food to eat in that company.

Poisoning with Crapaudin (Autopsy) (MIII,662)

M. de Castellan, King's Physician-in-Ordinary, (This was written in 1575, before M. de Castellan became Premier Physician of Catherine de' Médici.—Ed.) M. Jean d'Amboise, King's Surgeon-in-Ordinary and I were sent to open the body of a certain person suspected of having been poisoned, since before supper he had been well, not having any pain. Soon after supper he complained of a great pain in his stomach, crying that he was suffocating and his body became yellow and bloated. He could not get his breath, panting like a dog that had run hard, because the diaphragm (the chief instrument of respiration) could not move naturally, raced uncontrolled and hastened the rate of respiration. Then he developed vertigo, spasm, heart failure and consequently died.

Truly, the morning they showed us the corpse, it was swollen like a sheep inflated for the skinner. M. d'Amboise

made the first incision and I stepped back, sensing a stinking, cadaverous exhalation the assistants could hardly endure. The intestines and the internal parts in general were
inflated and filled with gas. We found a great quantity of
blood extending between the intestines and in the thoracic
cavity. It was concluded that the said person had been
poisoned with crapaudin.

Paré's Dissected Cadaver   (MIII,673)

I attest having a body given me after execution by the
Criminal Lieutenant. I dissected it twenty-five years or
more ago. (This must have been before 1550, probably
when he dissected with Thierry de Héry for the demon-
strations of the Faculty of Medicine.—ED.) I dissected
nearly all the muscles of the right side (so when I wanted
to make some incision, seeing the parts afresh made me
more sure in my work); the left side was left complete. To
preserve it better I punctured it in many places with a
punch to let the liquor penetrate deeply into the muscles
and other parts. Once can still see the entire lungs, heart,
diaphragm, stomach, spleen, kidneys. Similarly one can see
the hair of the beard, the head and other parts, the nails
which I have noticed grow evidently, after cutting them
several times.

Apology and Treatise, Containing the Voyages Made in Divers Places

THIS, the best known of Paré's writings, appeared in the fourth Edition of his Works in 1585. It was written in answer to a book by Étienne Gourmelen[127] published in 1580, attacking Paré for a number of his innovations. Those who have not done so are advised to read this delightful story, as much for insight into the life of his times as for accounts of his surgical experiences.

Histories of his cases are presented here in order of their appearance in the text. A few of them have been reported earlier in a little different detail.

Amputation of Leg with Ligatures
(MIII,681)

On June 16, 1582, in the presence of M. Jean Liébauld, Doctor of the Faculty of Medicine of Paris, Claude Viard,

---

[127] Born in Brittany, studied medicine in Paris, graduated March 5, 1561. He was appointed Dean of the Faculty 1574-1575 and Professor of Surgery of the Royal College by Henri III. He led the Faculty in a series of harassments of Paré for presuming to write in French on Surgery. In 1575 Paré published a tract addressed to the Court entitled *Response de A. P. Premier-Chirurgeon du Roi, aux calumnies d' Aucuns Médicins et Chirurgiens, touchant ses oeuvres*, etc. This is very rare, so was reprinted in toto by Le Paulmier (p. 223). In 1580, Gourmelen published a Surgery (*Chirurgicae artis, ex Hippocratis*, etc.) attacking Paré's new practices. He died at Melun on August 12, 1593 and is forgotten except as a stimulus for Paré to write his "Apologie and Treatise" in 1580, in which the now-mellowed old man ridiculed his opponent, "mon petit maitre," with barbed irony.

Licensed Surgeon, M. Mathurin Huron, Surgeon of M. de Souvray and me, Jean Charbonnel, Master Barber-Surgeon of Paris, well experienced in the theory and practice of Surgery, dextrously amputated the left leg of a woman. She had suffered more than three years of an extreme pain caused by extensive caries of the astragaloid and cuboid bones, the tibia and fibula and all the nervous parts, where she felt intolerable pain day and night. She was named Marie d'Hostel, aged about twenty-eight years, the wife of Pierre Herué, Esquire of the kitchen of Madame the Duchess of Uzés, living in the rue des Verbois beyond St. Martin-des-Champs, at the Sign of the Head of St. John. Charbonnel removed the leg four good inches below the knee.

After incising the flesh and sawing the bone, he caught the vein, then the artery with the crow's-beak (pincers —ED.) and then tied them. I declare to God (as the company present can testify) that during the entire, rapidly performed operation, not a pallet of blood was lost. I told Charbonnel to let more flow, following the precept of Hippocrates, that it is good to let blood flow in all wounds and inveterate ulcers, since thus the part is less subject to inflammation.

The said Charbonnel continued to dress and treat her, so she was healed in two months, without any hemorrhage, blood flow or other bad camplication. She went to see you in your house, being entirely cured.

Amputation of Leg, with Ligature
(MIII,682)

Another history of recent memory: M. Paulain, Chanter of Nôtre-Dame[128] broke the two bones of leg into several

---

[128] Nôtre-Dame (Cathedral). Probably the best known landmark in

fragments so there was no hope of healing. To avoid gangrene and mortification and consequent death, M. Helin, Regent Physician in the Faculty of Medicine, an honorable man of good knowledge, Claude Viard and Simon Piètre, Sworn Surgeons of Paris, men well practiced in Surgery and Balthasar de Lestre and Leonard de Leschenal, Master Barber-Surgeons, also well experienced in Surgical operations, agreed with me that to avoid the complications mentioned, the leg should be completely amputated a little above the broken and shattered bones and the lacerated nerves, veins and arteries.

The operation was dextrously performed by the said Viard and the blood stanched by ligature of the vessels, in the presence of the said Helin and of M. Tonsard, Grand Vicar of Nôtre-Dame. He was dressed continually by the said Leschenal and I visited him at times. He was happily cured without the application of hot irons, and walked gaily on a wooden leg.

Amputation of Leg, with Ligature
(MIII,682)

On December 10, 1583, Toussiant Posson, native of Roinville, living now at Beauvais near Dourdan, his leg all

---

Paris, the Cathedral on the Ile de la Cité was built and rebuilt on the site of an old Gallo-Roman temple. Construction of the present gothic structure was begun in 1163 and was largely finished under St. Louis in 1250, although additional minor work continued for another century. By the middle of the 18th century it had deteriorated badly and restoration begun by Viollet-le-Duc continued until the reign of Napoleon III (1864). In the 16th century the Hôtel-Dieu partly encroached on the view of its western facade, so after the hospital was burned in the 18th century, it was rebuilt in its present location across the island.

ulcerated and all the bone carious and purulent, begged me
that for the honor of God, I should cut off his leg because
of the great pain he could tolerate no longer. After preparing him, I had his leg cut off four fingers below the knee
cap by Daniel Poullet, one of my Assistants, to teach and
encourage him to do such work.

He tied the vessels very dextrously to stanch the blood,
without application of hot irons, in the presence of Jacques
Guillemeau, King's Surgeon-in-Ordinary, and Jean Charbonnel, Master Barber-Surgeon of Paris. During the cure
he was seen and examined by Messrs. Laffilé[129] and Courtin,
Regent Physicians in the Faculty of Medicine of Paris. The
operation was done in the house of Jean Gohel, Innkeeper
at the Sign of the White Horse in Gréve.

I do not want to forget here to say that Madame the
Princess of Montpensier,[130] knowing he was poor and in
my hands, gave him money to pay for his room and board.
He was well cured, thank God and returned to his home
with a wooden leg.

Leg Amputation for Gangrene, with Ligature (MIII,683)

Gangrene developed from an internal cause in half the
leg of sixty-six year old Nicholas Mesnager, living on rue
St. Honoré at the Sign of the Basket and we were constrained to amputate the leg to save his life. It was amputated by Antoine Renaud, Master Barber-Surgeon of Paris

---

[129] Pierre Lafillé, Bachelor in Medicine in 1550, Dean of the Faculty
in 1518-1519 (Sic?), died September 7, 1603 (Le Paulmier, p. 276).

[130] Probably the wife of Louise de Bourbon, Prince de Condé, who was
also duc de Montpensier.

the sixteenth day of December, 1583, in the presence of
Messrs. le Fort and La Noue,[131] Sworn Surgeons of Paris.
The blood was stanched by ligature of the vessels and he
is cured now, and in good health, walking with a wooden
leg.

Forearm Amputation, with Ligature
(MIII,683)

Jean Boussereau, a ferryman at the Port of Nesle, living
near Postmaster M. du Mats, had a harquebus burst in his
hand, breaking the bone and lacerating all the other parts
so it was necessary to amputate the hand two fingers above
the wrist. This was done by Jacques Guillemeau, at present
King's Surgeon-in-Ordinary, who then lived with me. The
operation also was done dextrously and the blood was
stanched by ligature of the vessels without the hot iron. He
is still living at present.

Ligature of Temporal Artery   (MIII,683)

A grocer merchant named le Juge, living on rue St. Denis
at the Sign of the Great Tournois fell on his head, causing
a wound near the temporal muscle. An artery was opened,
whence blood issued very impetuously so the remedies
commonly used to stanch it did not serve. I was called to

---

[131] Jerome was son of Mathurine de la Noüe, Surgeon of King Henri
II. He studied Medicine and Surgery, becoming Surgeon of Catherine
de' Médicis and of Kings Charles IX, Henri III and Henri IV. Licensed
to the Châtelet, he became Dean of the College of Surgeons and left
valuable historical references in their archives. He died February 17,
1628, leaving his posts and titles to his son Jean, who also became a
famous surgeon (Le Paulmier, p. 116).

stanch the blood and found Messrs. Rasse, Cointeret and Viard, Sworn Surgeons of Paris. I promptly took a threaded needle and tied the artery. It bled no more and he was soon healed. A witness would be M. Rousselet, recently Dean of your Faculty, who treated him with us.

Ligature of External Jugular Vein (MIII,683)

A Sergeant of the Châtelet, living near St. André-des-Arts, got a sword thrust in the throat in Pré-au-Clercs.[132] It cut the external jugular vein completely across. As soon as he was injured he put a handkerchief on the wound and came to my house to find me. When he removed the handkerchief blood flowed very freely. I immediately tied the vein toward its root; thus it was stanched and he recovered, thanks to God.

If you had followed your method of stanching the blood with cauteries, I wonder if he would have recovered. I believe he would have died in the hands of the operator.

Gunshot of Ankle, Captain le Rat (MIII,689)

(Action in Paré's first military expedition to Turin [Torino, Italy] in 1536, forcing the Pass of Suze, in the Piedmont Alps.—Ed.)

. . . but the enemy was constrained to retire and reached the Castle, which was taken partly by Captain le Rat, who with many soldiers of his company climbed a little mountain from which they shot down on the enemy. He received a

---

[132] The Pré-au-Clercs was a field outside the walls of the city in the Faubourgs-St. Germain between the Church of St. Germain-des-Prés and the Seine. In Paré's day it was a battle-ground for private duels and fights. Being convenient to his house, he treated many of the casualties.

harquebus shot in the right ankle. He fell instantly and cried, "At this hour the Rat is taken!" I dressed him and God healed him. (The first use in print of this famous phrase—ED.)

First Experience with Gunshot Wounds
(MIII,690)

The soldiers of the Castle (of Villaine—ED.), seeing our people coming in a tremendous fury, did everything possible to defend themselves, killing and wounding a great many of our soldiers with pike-thrusts and stones, giving the Surgeons a lot of work to do. I was at that time a little mild-of-salt (unseasoned—ED.) and had not yet seen the first dressing made in treating wounds made by harquebuses. It is true I had read in Jean de Vigo's first book "Wounds in General", Chapter 8, that wounds made by firearms were poisoned because of the powder. For their cure he advised their cauterization with boiling oil of Sambuc (elders—ED.) in which a little theriac is mixed. In order not to fail, before using the said oil, knowing such a thing could bring the patient severe pain, I wanted to know first how to apply it, what the other Surgeons did for the first dressing. They applied the said oil as hot as possible in the wounds with tents and setons. From this I took courage to do as they did.

Finally my oil ran out and I was constrained to apply as substitute a digestive made of egg yolk, rose oil and turpentine. That night I could not sleep at my ease, fearing that from failure to cauterize, I would find the wounded in whom I had failed to put the oil, dead of poisoning. This made me get up early to visit them, where beyond my hope, I found those on whom I had used the digestive mixture feeling little pain and their wounds neither inflamed nor swollen, having rested well enough through the night. The others to whom I had applied the said scalding oil, I found febrile, with great pain and swelling around their wounds. Then I resolved never again so cruelly to burn the poor victims of gun fire. (See also pg. 57—Ed.)

Experience in Garrison (MIII,691)

The said Seigneur le Maréschal de Montejan remained in Piedmont as King's Lieutenant-General, having 10-12,000 men in garrison among the towns and Châteaux. These often fought among themselves with swords and other weapons and even firearms, and if four were wounded, I always had three of them. If it was a question of amputating an arm or a leg, or trepanning, or reducing a fracture or dislocation, I took care of it. My Lord the Maréschal sent me sometime to one place, sometime to another to treat special soldiers, who were fighting in other towns as much as at Turin, so I was always in the field in one place or another.

Death of Wrestler in Low-Brittany (MIII,693)

At other times he had wrestlers come from towns and villages where they had taken prizes. The game rarely ended without someone having an arm or leg broken or a shoulder or hip dislocated.

There was one little low-Breton, well set up, solid and muscled, who for a long time held the field and by his skill and strength threw five or six. Then came Dativo, a big schoolmaster, said to be one of the best wrestlers in Brittany. He entered the lists, having removed his long jacket, in hose and doublet and standing near the little man he looked as if he had been tied to his belt to prevent him from running. Nevertheless when they gripped collar to collar, for a long time they did nothing, appearing to equal skill and strength. But the little one hurled himself in an ambling jerk under the big Dativo, charged him with his shoulder and threw him to earth on his back, sprawled like a frog. Then everybody began laughing at the strength and skill of the little fellow. The big Dativo was furious at having been thrown by such a little man. He sprang up angrily and demanded his revenge. They went again collar to collar and again were a long time at their hold, neither able to throw the other. Finally this huge man let himself fall on the little one and in the fall put his elbow into the pit of his stomach, ruptured his heart and killed him stark dead. Knowing he had given him the death blow, he took his long jacket and went with his tail between his legs and disappeared. Seeing that the little man's heart did not recover after wine, vinegar or anything else given him, I approached him, tested the pulse which did not beat, then said that he was dead. Then the Bretons who assisted at the wrestling, shouted in their jabbering, that is not in the Sport. Someone said that the big Dativo was accustomed to doing this and that only a year before he had done the same in wrestling.

I wanted to open the corpse to find what had caused this sudden death. I found much blood spread from the thorax to the lower belly and I tried hard to find some opening through which so much blood could have passed, but I could not find it, for all the care I used. But I believe it was by diapedesis or anastomosis, that is to say, by the openings of the mouths of the vessels, or by their porosities. The poor little wrestler was buried.

Gunshot Wound of Shoulder. Location of Missile   (MIII,694)

. . . very many were killed and wounded (at Perpignan, 1545—Ed.), among others M. de Brissac (then Grand Master of Artillery—Ed.) of a harquebus shot in the shoulder. On returning to his tent, all the wounded followed him, hoping to be treated by the Surgeons coming to dress him. Having reached his tent and been put on his bed, the ball was searched for by three or four of the most expert Surgeons of the Army who could not find it, saying it had entered his body. Finally he called me to know if I could be more fortunate than they, for he had known me in Piedmont. At once I had him get out of bed and told him he should put himself in the same position as he was when wounded. This he did and took a javelin in his hands just as he then had held a pike for fighting. I put my hand near the wound and found the ball in the flesh making a little tumor under the shoulder blade. Having found it, I showed the spot and it was removed by M. Nicole Lavernault.[132a] Surgeon of M. le Dauphin (later Henri II—Ed.) who was the King's Lieutenant in this Army. I still retained the honor of having found it. (See also pg. 60—Ed.)

Brain Wound with Preservation of Consciousness   (MIII,695)

I saw a very remarkable thing (in the camp at Perpignan —Ed.). It was that in my presence a soldier struck one of his companions on the head with a halberd penetrating the

[132a] Nicolle Lavernot, a Surgeon of King François I and of Henri the Dauphin, later of King Henri II and finally Premier-Surgeon of Charles IX. He died in this post in 1561 and Paré replaced him on January 1, 1562. He had been one of the officials of the College of Surgeons when Paré was admitted to membership in 1554.

left ventricle of the brain without knocking him down. The one who struck him said he had cheated at dice and had taken a large sum of money, and was accustomed to cheat. They asked me to dress him, which I did to acquit my conscience, knowing quite well he would die. Having been dressed, he returned alone to his lodging, which was at least two hundred paces away. I told one of his companions that they should call a Priest to arrange the affairs of his soul. He called one who remained with him to his last breath. The next day the patient sent for me by his girl dressed as a boy, to dress him. I did not want to do it, fearing he would die in my hands. To put it off I told him his dressing should not be changed until the third day, since he would die without touching it again. On the third day be came staggering into my tent to find me, accompanied by his wench and begged me fondly to dress him. He showed me a purse where he had a hundred to one hundred twenty gold pieces and told me he would pay me what I wanted. Despite all that, I delayed changing his dressing, fearing he would die instantly. Certain Gentlemen requested me to go dress him, which I did at their request, but during the dressing, he died in my hands in convulsions.

But the Priest who stayed with him till death took his purse, fearing someone else would take it, saying he would say masses for his poor soul. In addition, he seized his clothes and all his other possessions.

I have recited this history as a monstrous thing, that the soldier, having received this great blow, did not fall down and was rational until death.

Wound by Concussion by Passing Cannonball (MIII,696)

One day, going by the camp (before Boulogne, 1545 —Ed.) to treat my wounded, the enemy in the tower ordered firing a piece of artillery, thinking to kill two men-at-arms who had stopped to talk together. The ball happened to pass very near one of them, throwing him to the ground, making one think the ball had struck him. It had not at all, but only the wind of the said ball in the middle of his tassette (thigh-armor—Ed.), which had such force that all the external surface of the thigh became livid and black. He could hardly stand because of the extreme pain. I treated him and made several incisions to evacuate the bruised blood caused by the blast of the ball. And in the bounces it made on the ground, four soldiers were killed on the spot.

I was not far from this shot and felt some of the agitation of the air. This did me no harm except fear making me bow my head very low, but the ball was already far away.

Lance Wound, Duc de Guise   (MIII,696)

M. le duc de Guise, François de Lorraine, was wounded before Boulogne by a lance stroke which passed from over his right eye, declined toward the nose, entered and passed out the other side between the ear and the neck. The force was so great that the iron lance tip, with a portion of the wood was broken off and remained imbedded. It was impossible to pull it out except with great force, using a blacksmith's tongs. Notwithstanding such great violence, which fractured bones, tore and lacerated nerves, veins, arteries and other parts, my said Lord, by the grace of God, recovered.

This Knight always went into a fight with his face uncovered, which is why the lance passed through the other side. (See also pg. 27—Ed.)

Treatment of Army Servant in Ambulance
(MIII,697)

(Expedition to Germany, Toul and Metz, 1552—Ed.)
One of the servants of a Captain assigned to the Company of M. de Rohan[133] went with others intending to enter a church where the peasants had retreated, thinking to find food by love or by force. But among others, he was well beaten and returned with seven sword cuts on the head, the least penetrating to the second table of the skull. He had four others in the arms and one on the right shoulder which cut more than half the shoulder blade, or scapula. He was brought to the lodge of his Master, who seeing him so wounded, and since we had to leave at daybreak tomorrow, thinking he could never recover, had a grave made and would have thrown him into it, saying that was better than have the peasants massacre and kill him.

Moved by pity I told him he still might recover if he was dressed well. Many Gentlemen of the Company begged him to have him brought with the baggage, since I had thus volunteered to treat him. This he granted and after I dressed him, he was put well covered and accommodated on a bed in a cart drawn by one horse. I did him the services of Physician, Apothecary, Surgeon and cook. I treated him to the end of his cure and God healed him. All those of three Companies praised this cure. At the first muster that was made the men-at-arms of M. de Rohan's Company each gave me a crown and the archers a half-crown.

---

[133] Vicomte de Rohan, Comte de Porrhoët and de la Garnache, de Beauvoir-sur-Mer and of Carentan, Prince de Léon. In 1534, married Isabelle d'Albret, daughter of Jean, King of Navarre and sister of Antoine de Bourbon. He was Paré's second Master-at-war, to whom Paré dedicated his book on "Anatomy" in 1549. He was killed on November 4, 1552 at St. Nicholas, near Nancy.

Leg Amputation with Ligature   (MIII,698)

Returning from the German camp, King Henry besieged Damvilliers (July 1, 1552—Ed.) and the inhabitants would not surrender. They were well beaten when our powder failed, during which they shot several of our people. A culverin shot passed through the tent of M. de Rohan striking the leg of a Gentleman of his Company. It was necessary that I finish removing it, which was done without using the hot irons.

The camp broken up, . . . I returned to Paris with my Gentleman whose leg I had amputated: I dressed him and God healed him. I returned him to his house, merry with a wooden leg and he was content, saying he had got off cheaply for not have been miserably burned to stanch the blood, as you write in your book, my little Master. (Gourmelen—Ed.)

(This is Paré's first recorded report of reliance on ligature to control hemorrhage in amputations. See also pg. 73 —Ed.)

Neglected Fractured Leg   (MIII,701)

M. le Prince de la Roche-sur-Yon was the first to feast me (after his entry into besieged Metz) and he inquired what was said at the Court of the City of Metz. I told him as much as I wished. Then he asked me to go see one of his Gentlemen, named M. de Magnane, at present Chevalier of the Order of the King and Lieutenant of His Majesty's Guards, whose leg was broken by a cannon shot.

I found him in bed, his leg crooked and bent without any dressing on it, because a gentleman had promised him a cure with certain words, having taken his name and girdle.

And the poor Gentleman wept and cried with the pain he felt, sleeping neither day nor night for four days. Then I mocked at this imposture and false promise. I promptly set and dressed his leg so dextrously that he was free of pain and slept all night. He since was cured, thanks to God, and is still living and serving the King. The said Seigneur de la Roche-sur-Yon sent a cask of wine larger than a pipe of Anjou to my lodgings and told me that when it was drunk he would send me another. That was how he treated me, making me very happy.

Frontal Depressed Fracture, Trepanned (Metz, 1552—Ed.)   (MIII,702)

All the besieged Lords prayed me to treat more carefully than all the others, M. de Pienne, who was wounded on the breach (of the city wall—Ed.) by a stone cannon ball in the temple with fracture and depression of the bone. They told me that immediately on receiving the wound he fell to earth as though dead, bleeding from the mouth, nose and ears, with profuse vomiting and for fourteen days had been speechless and irrational. Also he had developed jerking resembling convulsions and his face was swollen and livid. He was trepanned at the side of the temporal muscle on the frontal bone. I dressed him with other Surgeons and God healed him. Today he is still living, thank God. (See also pg. 36—Ed.)

Fatal Shoulder Cannon Shot   (MIII,710)

The duc Horace[134] got a cannon shot to one shoulder which carried away his arm in one direction and his body

---

[134] Horace Farnese, duc de Castro, was one of the nobles besieged at Metz to whom Paré brought personal greetings from the King. After

in another, without being able to say a single word. His death to us was a great disaster, for the rank he held in this place.(At the siege of Hesdin, 1543—ED.)

Chest Wound, Fatal. Autopsy   (MIII,710)

Similarly, M. de Martigues was struck by a bullet that pierced his lungs. I treated him, as I will describe later (see also pg. 9 and 68). (As the castle was to be surrendered, Paré exchanged clothing with a dirty soldier for disguise, in an attempt to escape being held for ransom—ED.)

I went in this makeup to M. de Martigues, whom I prayed that he order me to remain behind to dress him; this he granted me quite willingly. He wanted me to remain with him as much as I did. . . .

But to return to my story, as I was taken from the Castle into the town with M. de Martigues, a Gentleman of M. de Savoy asked me if M. de Martigues' wound could be cured. I told him no and that it was incurable. Promptly he went to tell this to M. the Duke de Savoy. I thought he would sent his Physicians and Surgeons to examine and treat M. de Martigues. In the meantime I considered in my mind if I should play the fool and not reveal myself as a Surgeon for fear they would keep me to treat their wounded, and in the end if I was recognized as a Surgeon of the King, they would make me pay a big ransom. On the other hand, I feared that if I did not show myself as a Surgeon and had dressed M. de Martigues well, they would cut my throat. So I resolved to let them know that he would not die from failure of having been well dressed and looked after.

---

returning to Paris, he married the King's "natural" daughter, Diane d' Angoulême. From his honeymoon he went with the relief force to Hesdin, where in the siege in July, 1553, he was killed by a cannon shot.

Soon after, I saw many Gentlemen coming, accompanied
by a Physician and a Surgeon of the Emperor and those of
the said Duke de Savoy, with six other Surgeons following
the Army, to see the wound of M. de Martigues and to find
out from me how I had dressed and treated him. The Emperor's Physician told me I should declare the essence of
the wound and how I treated it. But all the Assistants had
their ears open to know if the wound was mortal or not.

I began by telling them that M. de Martigues, looking
from the top of the wall to reconnoiter those who were
sapping it, received a harquebus shot through the body,
after which I was called to treat him. I saw that he bled
from the mouth and from his wounds. Moreover, he had
great difficulty breathing and expelled air by the wounds,
with a whistling that would have blown out a candle, saying he had severe stabbing pain where the ball had entered.
I think and believe that there could be some bone fragments
that pricked the lungs when they make their systole and
diastole. I put my finger in, where I found that the entry
of the ball had broken the fourth rib in its middle and some
spicules the said ball had pushed in. In emerging, it had
similarly broken the fifth rib, with spicules that had been
driven from within outward. I took some of them out, but
not all, since they were too deep and adherent. I put in
each wound a tent with a large head, attached by a thread,
for fear that with inspiration they might be drawn into the
cavity of the thorax, which has been known by experience,
to the detriment of the poor wounded. For, having fallen in
one cannot remove them, causing them to engender a putrefaction, as a thing foreign to nature. The said tents were
anointed with a medication made of egg yolks and Venice
turpentine, with a little oil of roses. My purpose in placing
the tents was to stop the bleeding and to prevent the ex-

ternal air from entering the chest, which could cool the
lungs and consequently the heart. The said tents were
placed also to give issue to blood spilled in the thorax. I put
on the wounds a great diachalciteos plaster in which I had
mixed rose oil and vinegar to prevent inflammation. Then
afterward I put large compresses wet with oxycrat and
bandaged him, not too tightly so he could breathe easily.
This done, I drew five pallets of blood from the basilic vein
of the right arm, to make revulsion of blood which escaped
from the wounds into the thorax, having first taken into account the parts wounded and chiefly his strength, considering his youth and his sanguine temperament. Soon afterward he went to his affairs, passing a great deal of blood in
his urine and stool. And as for the pain he suffered at the
wound of entrance, as if he had been stabbed with a dagger,
that was caused by the lungs, in their movements, beating
against the spicules of the broken rib. The lungs are covered
by a tunic coming from the pleural membrane supplied by
nerves of the sixth pair from the brain, which was cause for
the pain he felt.

Also he had great difficulty inhaling and exhaling, which
was due to blood poured into the thoracic cavity and in the
diaphragm, chief muscle of respiration, and to laceration of
muscles on each side, which also assist in making inspiration
and expiration; likewise the lungs were torn, broken and
lacerated by the ball, which has made him spit up black
putrid blood when coughing.

He developed fever soon after he was hurt with failure
of the heart. This fever seemed to me to develop from
putrid vapors arising from the blood that is out of its vessels, which flows and will continue to flow. The wound of
the lung is large and will enlarge more, since it is in constant motion whether he is asleep or awake and they dilate

and contract to draw the air to the heart and to expel
fuliginous vapors. Inflammation develops from the unnatu-
ral heat; then the expulsive force attempts to throw out
what is harmful. But the lung can purge itself only by
coughing, and in coughing the wound dilates further and
grows constantly, causing blood to flow in larger amount,
which blood is drawn from the heart by the arterial vein to
nourish them, and to the heart from the vena cava.

His diet was barley broth, prunes with sugar, at other
times of bread soup; his drink was of infusion of herbs. He
could lie only on his back, which shows him to have a great
volume of blood spilled into the thoracic cavity and extending along the spine, not compressing the lungs as much as
if he lay on the side or sat up.

What more can I say? Only that since he was wounded,
M. de Martigues has not known a single hour of rest and
always passes bloody stools and urine. These things considered, Messieurs, one can make no other prognosis than
that he will die in a few days, which is with my profound
regret.

Having delivered my discourse I dressed him in my
usual manner. Having uncovered his wounds, the Physicians and Surgeons and other Assistants present knew the
truth of what I had said. The Physicians felt the pulse and
knew his strength to be almost spent and beaten, concluded
with me that he would die in a few days. With that they returned to the Duke de Savoy and told him M. de Martigues
would die in a short time. He replied that possibly if he had
been well dressed he might have recovered. Then all with
one voice told him that he had been very well dressed and
cared for in every possible way, and the treatment of his
wounds could not have been better. It was impossible to
cure him and his wound was necessarily mortal. Then the

Duke de Savoy showed great displeasure and wept (probably more from loss of a rich ransom than from friendship!
—Ed.) and demanded afresh if they were certain that all
was lost. They answered yes.

Intrusion of an Imposter. Then a Spanish imposter presented himself and promised on his life to cure him, and
if he failed to cure him they should cut him into a hundred
pieces. He did not want to have any Physicians, Surgeons
nor Apothecaries with him. At once the Duke de Savoy told
the Physicians and Surgeons that they should not go see
the said M. de Martigues again. Also he sent a Gentleman
to guard me, on pain of life, of not touching M. de Martigues again. This I promised to do, very gladly, seeing that
he would not die in my hands. He commanded this imposter to treat the said M. de Martigues and that he should
have no other Physician nor Surgeon than himself.

He came to M. de Martigues at once and told him:
"Senor Caballero, M. le Duc de Savoy has commanded me
to take over the treatment of your wound. I swear to God
that within eight days I will have you on horseback, lance
in hand, provided that no one but myself touches you. You
will eat and drink what pleases you; I will diet for you, on
that I give you my promise. I have cured many having
greater wounds than yours."

And the Lord replied, "God give you the grace to do it."

He demanded one of M. de Martigues' shirts and he
tore it into little strips which he lay on the wounds in form
of a cross, mumbling and babbling certain words. Having
dressed him he let him eat and drink what he wished, telling him he would diet for him. This he did, eating only six
prunes and six morsels of bread for repast, drinking only
some beer. Nevertheless, Sr. de Martigues died and my
Spaniard, seeing him in agony, disappeared and got away

without saying adieu to anyone. I believe that if he had been caught he would have been hanged for the false promise he made to M. le Duc de Savoy and several other Gentlemen.

He died at ten o'clock in the morning and in the afternoon the Seigneur de Savoy sent his Physicians and Surgeons and his Apothecary, with a quanty of drugs to embalm him. They came accompanied by many Gentlemen and Captains of the Army.

The Emperor's Surgeon approached me and kindly asked me to open the body. This I refused, protesting that I did not merit carrying his case after him. He prayed me again that I do it for his friendship, and he was very agreeable. I wished again to excuse myself and since he did not want to do it, he should give the duty to another Surgeon in the company. He again replied that he wished me to do it, and if I would not, I might well repent it. Knowing this particular affection, for fear he would do me some displeasure, I took the razor and presented it to all in particular, protesting to them that I was not well practiced in doing such an operation. They all refused it.

Autopsy: The body placed on a table, truly I decided to show them that I was an Anatomist, declaring to them too many things to recite here. I began by saying to all the Company that I was sure the ball had broken two ribs and had passed through the lungs, and that their wound would be found greatly enlarged, since they are in constant motion while sleeping or awake. By this motion the wound tears itself larger, so a great quantity of blood would be spilled in the chest and on the diaphragm. And some spicules of the rib fractures would be found, that entry of the ball had pushed in and the exit had pushed out. Indeed, all I told them was found in the dead body.

One of the Physicians asked me how the blood contained in the thorax could pass to be expelled through the urine. I replied that it had a manifest conduit: this was the azygos vein; having nourished all the ribs, the remainder descends under the diaphragm. On the left side it joints the emulgent vein, which is the way by which the matter of pleurisy and the pus of empyemas manifestly empty themselves in the urine and the stool.—(A tortured bit of patho-physiology resulting from ignorance of the circulation of the blood. —Ed.)

Our discourse finished, I embalmed the body and it was put in a coffin.

Cure of Leg Ulcer (Varicose)   (MIII,716)

M. de Vaudeville,[135] Governor of Graveline and Colonel of sixteen ensigns of Infantry prayed him (Duc de Savoy, after capture of Paré at Hesdin, 1553—Ed.) to give me to him to treat an old ulcer he had had on one of his legs for six or seven years. M. de Savoy told him that for all I was worth, he was content and that if I put fire to his leg, it would be done well. He replied that if he noticed any such thing he would have my throat cut.

Soon afterward the said Lord of Vaudeville sent for me with four German halberdies of his guard. This frightened me badly, not knowing where they took me; they spoke no more French than I German. Having arrived at his place, he told me I was welcome and that I belonged to him. He told me that if I could cure an ulcer he had on his leg, he would set me free without taking any ransom from me. I told him I had no means of paying any ransom.

---

[135] Vandeville—Governor of Graavelines, a village between Calais and Dunkerque. Served with the Imperial forces at Hesdin.

Then he called his Physician and Surgeon-in-Ordinary to show me the leg ulcer. Having seen and considered it, we retired apart in a chamber, where I began to tell them that the said ulcer was annular, was not simple but complicated, that is, of a round contour and scaly, having hard, calloused borders, concave and dirty, accompanied by a large varicose vein that perpetually irrigated it. Moreover, there was a great swelling and phlegmonous, painful distemper in the whole leg, in a strongly choleric body, as the hair, the beard and the face revealed.

The method of curing it, if it could be cured, required beginning with basic things, that is, with purgations, bleedings and the matter of diet. He should use no wine, nor salt nor highly seasoned foods, those things in general that heat the blood. Afterward, it was necessary to being the cure by making several scarifications around the said ulcer, remove the callous border and give it a long or triangular figure. For the round ones can heal only difficultly, as the ancients have written and as can be seen by experience. That done, it was necessary to cleanse the sordid and putrid flesh of the ulcer with Egyptiac ointment and over it a compress treated with juice of plantain, nightshade and oxycrat. One must bandage his leg, commencing at the foot and finishing at the knee and not forget to put a little compress on the varicose vein so it can bring nothing superfluous to the said ulcer. Moreover, that he keep himself in repose on the bed, as Hippocrates recommended, saying that those who have bad legs should not remain standing nor sitting, but reclining. After these things are done and the ulcer well cleansed, one should apply to it a lead plate rubbed and whitened with mercury. Those are the means by which the said Seigneur de Vaudeville could be cured of this ulcer.

All of this they found good. Then the Physician left me

with the Surgeon and going to M. de Vaudeville, told him
he was sure I could cure him and told him all I had planned
to do to heal his ulcer, which made him very happy. He had
me called and asked me if I believed I could cure his ulcer.
I told him yes, provided he was obedient to do what he
should. He promised me he would do entirely what I
wished and ordered for him and that as soon as the ulcer
was healed he would give me liberty to return without paying any ransom. Then I begged him to come to a better
bargain with me, protesting that the time would be too long
before being free if I stayed with him until he was entirely
cured. In fifteen days I hoped to make his ulcer shrink more
than half and be painless, and his Surgeon and Physician
quite easily could finish what remained. He agreed to this
and then I took a piece of paper to take the size of his ulcer.
I gave this to him and kept a similar one for myself. I
prayed him that he keep his promise when he knew the job
was done. He swore me his faith as a Gentleman that he
would do it. Then I resolved to dress him well, after the
method of Galen which was that after having removed the
foreign things from the ulcer, only rebuilding the flesh was
required.

I dressed him only once a day, which he found strange,
as did his Physician, who was fresh at these things and
wished with the patient to persuade me to dress him two or
three times a day. I prayed them to let me alone and that
what I did was not to prolong the cure; on the contrary, to
shorten it, for the desire I had to be free, etc.—then the
said Seigneur de Vaudeville did not want to be dressed
more than once a day. So, within fifteen days his ulcer was
nearly all cicatrized. The contract between us being filled, I
began to enjoy myself. He made me eat and drink at his
table when there were no men of higher rank present.

He gave me a great red scarf that he ordered me to wear. I can say I was as happy with it as a dog to which one ties a clog for fear he will go to the vines to eat the grapes. The Physician and Surgeon took me through the Camp to visit their wounded, where I noticed what our enemies did. I saw they had no great pieces of battery, but only twenty-five or thirty for the field. . . .

And to return to my story, soon after my said Lord de Vaudeville was very well and his ulcer was nearly healed, so he gave me my freedom and had me conducted with a passport and a trumpet to Abbeville. There I took the post and went to find King Henry, my Master, at Aufimon. He received me with joy and with good grace.

Quartan Fever Broken by Neck Wound
(MIII,722)

. . . they killed and wounded many of our Captains and good soldiers (at Dourlan, near Amiens, 1558—Ed.) and among others the Captain St. Aubin, valiant with the sword, whom M. de Guise loved greatly, and for whom chiefly the King sent me there. When he was in an attack of quartan fever he wilfully set out to lead the greater part of his company. A Spaniard, seeing that he commanded, perceived him to be a Captain and shot a harquebus-bullet through his neck. My Captain St. Aubin thought himself dead of the shot, and from the fear, I protest to God, he lost his quartan fever and was freed of it entirely. (See also pg. 6—Ed.) I dressed him with Antoine Portail, King's Surgeon-in-Ordinary, and many other soldiers. Some died, others escaped, relieved of an arm or a leg, or loss of an eye; and those say they got off lightly: escape who can. When the enemy broke camp, I returned to Paris. Here I will say nothing

of my little Master, who had more ease in his house than
I at the war.

Bullet in Cavity of Humerus   (MIII,723)

The King of Navarre was wounded some days after the
assault (on Rouen, October 26, 1562—Ed.) by a bullet
wound of the shoulder. I visited him and helped dress him
with one of his Surgeons, M. Gilbert, one of the best of
Montpellier and others. The ball could not be found. I
searched for it very exactly. I decided by conjecture that it
had entered by the head of the humerus, and had run down
the cavity of the bone, hence could not be found. The ma-
jority said it had entered and been lost in the body. M. le
Prince de la Roche-sur-Yon, who intimately loved the
King of Navarre, drew me apart and inquired if the wound
was mortal. I told him yes, since all wounds of major joints,
and especially contused wounds are mortal, according to all
authors who have written on them. He asked the others
what they thought and especially the said Gilbert, who told
him he had great hope his Master the King would recover,
and the said Prince was very happy. Four days later watching us dress the King of Navarre, the King (Charles IX—
Ed.) and the Queen-Mother, M. the Prince de la Roche-
sur-Yon, M. de Guise and other Great People, wanted a
consultation held in their presence, where there were many
Physicans and Surgeons. Each said what he believed, and
they all had good hope the King would recover, but I persisted to the contrary. M. the Prince de la Roche-sur-Yon,
who loved me, took me aside and told me I was alone
against so many good men. I told him that when I recognized good signs of improvement I would change my advice. Many consultations were held, where I never changed

my word and prognosis made at the first dressing and always said the arm would fall into gangrene. This it did, despite the greatest care possible to make, and he gave up his spirit to God on the eighteenth day of his wound.

Autopsy: M. the Prince de la Roche-sur-Yon, having told the King of his death, sent his Surgeon and Physician named le Fèvre, at present Physician-in-Ordinary to the King and the Queen-Mother, to me to tell me he wanted to have the ball and that they should search out its location. Then I was happy and told them I was sure of finding it quickly. This I did in their presence and that of many Gentlemen: it was in the very center of the cavity of the humerus. The Prince took it and showed it to the King and the Queen-Mother who told everyone my prognosis had been proved correct. The body was laid to rest at the Château Gaillard[136] and I returned to Paris. There I found many patients who had been wounded at the breach at Rouen.

Pistol Wound of Femur (MIII,724)

The day after the battle given at Dreux (on December 19, 1562—ED.), the King commanded me to go treat M. the Comte d'Eu,[137] who had been wounded by a pistol shot

---

[136] Château Gaillard, an interesting ruin now at les Andelys on the Seine, 92 Km. from Paris, of a huge castle built in 1197 by Richard the Lion-Hearted, duc de Normandy and King of England. Considered impregnable, it fell to the attack of Philippe-August seven years later, after the death of Richard removed its valiant defender.

[137] François de Cleves, Duc de Nevers, Comte d' Auxerre, de Rethel and of d'Eu Seigneur d' Orval; Governor of Champagne, born in 1539. He married 1) Anne de Bourbon and 2) Jacquelin de Longwic. He commanded the French Army assembled at Laon before the battle of St. Quentin. Before the battle of Dreux (December 12, 1562) he was shot by accident by one of his Gentlemen and, as Paré said, the wound was fatal (Paget, 147).

in the right thigh near the hip joint, which had fractured and broken the femur into many fragments, from which numerous complications developed, then he died. This gave me profound regret.

Conditions of Military Surgery, 1562
(MIII,724)

In the meantime while at Dreux I visited and dressed a great number of Gentlemen and poor soldiers, and among others, many Swiss Captains. I dressed fourteen of them in a single room, all wounded with shots of pistols and other diabolical fire arms, and not one of the fourteen died. M. le Comte d'Eu being dead, I tarried no longer at Dreux. Surgeons came from Paris to do their duty to the wounded, such as Pigray, Cointeret, Hubert and others. I returned to Paris where I found many wounded Gentlemen who had retired after the said battle to have their wounds dressed.

(Surgeons were now going to the battle fields. Paré had made Military Surgery "respectable."—Ed.)

Conditions of Military Surgery, 1569
(MIII,725)

During the battle of Montcontour (October 3, 1569—Ed.) King Charles was at Plessis-lès-Tours,[138] where he heard of the victory. A great number of wounded Gentlemen and soldiers retired into the city and suburbs of towns to be dressed and treated. The King and the Queen-Mother ordered me to do my duty, with the other Surgeons then in

---

[138] A chateau 3 Km. east of Tours built by Louis XI, who died there in 1483.

the area, such as Pigray, du Bois, Portail and one named
Siret, a Surgeon of Tours, a man well learned in Surgery,
then Surgeon of Monseigneur,[139] brother of the King.
From the number of wounded, we had little rest, nor the
Physicians either.

Gunshot Wounds of Elbow   (MIII,725)

M. le Comte de Mansfeld, Governor of the Duchy of
Luxembourg, Chevalier of the Order of the King of Spain,
was gravely wounded at the battles (Moncontour, October
3, 1569—Ed.), in the left arm by a pistol shot which broke
a large part of the elbow joint; he had retired to Bourgueil,[140] near Tours. Being there, he sent a Gentleman to
the King, begging him affectionately to send one of his
Surgeons to help him with his wound. A Council was held
to decide which Surgeon to send him. M. le Maréschal de
Montmorency told the King and Queen that it would be
well to send his Premier Surgeon, reminding them that the
said Seigneur de Mansfeld had had a great part in winning
the battle. The King said flatly that he did not want me to

---

[139] Herculé, François, duc d'Alencon (Anjou) (1555-1584), fifth son
of Henri II and Catherine de' Médicis. He was the last of the Valois
heirs during the life of Henri III and had ambitions to succeed or to
displace his brother. A favorite of his mother, he was difficult to govern
and turned Huguenot. In 1581 he seized control of Holland as duc de
Brabant and Comte de Flandres and tried to capture Antwerp, but was
repulsed. Returning to France in 1584 he was reconciled to Henri III,
but died suddenly of pulmonary hemorrhage at Château Thierry on
June 10, 1584.

[140] Bourgueil, a town near Tours, to which many retreated after
being wounded at the battle of Moncontour October 3, 1569. At the
request of the Comte de Mansfeld, Paré was sent there by the King to
treat him. Paré worked there for three weeks with Portail, Pigray,
DuBois and other colleagues.

go and wanted me to remain with him. Then the Queen-Mother told him I could go and return; that he must remember that this was a foreign Lord, who had come to his assistance on behalf of the King of Spain. Then he let me go, provided I returned quickly.

Then he and the Queen-Mother sent for me and ordered me to go find the said Comte de Mansfeld wherever he might be, to serve him and do all I could to cure his wound. I went to find him, carrying a letter from their Majesties. Having seen it, he received me with good will and released three or four Surgeons who had dressed him. I regretted this greatly, since the wound appeared incurable to me.

Now at Bourgueil were many Gentlemen who had retired there after being wounded in the said battle, knowing that M. de Guise was there. He had been badly hurt by a pistol shot through a leg and they knew well he would have good Surgeons to treat him. They also knew he was kind and very generous and would help them in many of their necessities. This he did willingly, for their food and drink as well as for other necessities. For my part they were helped and aided by my Art; some died, others lived, according to their wounds. The Comte Ringrave died: he had a shoulder wound like that of the King of Navarre before Rouen. M. de Bassompierre, Colonel of 1200 Horse, was wounded by a blow like that of M. le Comte de Mansfeld, whom I dressed and God healed (See pg. 63—Ed.). God so well blessed my work that in three weeks I took them to Paris where it was necessary to make some additional incisions in the arm of the Comte de Mansfeld to remove the bone that was badly fractured, broken and carious. He recovered, by the grace of God and gave me an honest reward, so I was as well pleased with him as he was with me, as he subsequently showed me. (See also pg. 60—Ed.)

He wrote a letter to M. the Duc d'Ascot telling how he was cured of his wound, as was also M. de Bassompierre of a similar one, and many others wounded after the battle of Moncontour. He advised him to request the King of France to permit me to go see his brother, M. le Marquis d'Auret, which he did.

Gunshot Wound of Knee—Complicated (MIII,726)

M. le Duc d'Ascot sent a Gentleman to the King (Charles IX—Ed.) with a letter humbly begging him to do him the honor and favor of permitting and commanding his Premier Surgeon to go see his brother, the Marquis d'Auret. He had received a harquebus shot near the knee, with fracture of the bone about seven months earlier that the neighborhood Physicians and Surgeons had been unable to cure. The King sent for me and ordered me to go see the said M. d'Auret and to help him all I could to cure his wound. I told him I would use all the little knowledge God had been pleased to give me.

Conducted by the two Gentlemen (Autumn, 1569—Ed.) I went to the Château d'Auret, about a league and a half from Mons in Heinaut, where the Marquis was. As soon as I arrived I visited him and told him the King had commanded me to come to see him and dress his wound. He told me he was very joyful for my visit and was greatly indebted to the King who had done him the honor to send me to him.

I found him with a high fever, the eyes deeply sunken, with a yellow, moribund face, the tongue dry and rough, his whole body thin and emaciated, his voice low, like that of a man very near death. Then I found his thigh very swollen, purulent and ulcerated, draining a green and strongly fetid pus. I probed it with a silver sound. Thus I found a cavity near the groin ending in the middle of the thigh and others around the knee sanious and channelled; also certain splinters of bone, some separated, others not. The leg was greatly enlarged and filled with a phlegmy humor, cold, humid and flatulent (to the degree that the natural heat was on the way to being suffocated and extinguished). It was bent and retracted toward the buttock, the rump ulcerated to the size of the palm of a hand. He said he felt an extreme burning and pain, in his flanks as well, so he could take no rest day or night, and he had no appetite to eat, but enough to drink. I was told that he often fell fainting and sometimes as if in epilepsy. He often wanted to vomit, with such tremors that he could not carry his hands to his mouth.

Seeing and considering all these serious complications, and the great weakening of his strength, truly I had a great regret of having come to him, for he seemed to me to have little evidence that he could escape death. Nevertheless, to give him courage and good hope, I told him that soon I would put him on his feet, by the Grace of God and the help of his Physician and Surgeon. Having seen him, I went to walk in a garden, where I prayed God that he grant me this favor, that he recover and that he bless our hands and the medications to combat such complicated maladies. I went over in my mind the means I must take to do it. They called me to dinner; I entered the kitchen where I saw drawn from a huge cauldron a half sheep, a quarter of veal, three big pieces of beef, two pullets, and a big side of bacon, with a lot of good vegetables. Then I said to myself that this hot bouillon was succulent and very nourishing.

After dinner all the Physicians and Surgeons assembled and we went into conference in the presence of M. le Duc d'Ascot and some Gentlemen who accompanied him. I began by telling the Surgeons I marvelled greatly that they had not opened M. le Marquis' thigh, which was all abscessed and since the pus that drained was strongly fetid and stinking, which shows it to have been long confined and that with the sound I found caries of the bone and spicules that had separated. They replied he never would consent and that for nearly two months they had not been able to change the sheets of his bed and hardly dared to touch the counterpaine, since it hurt him so much. Then I said that to cure him it would be necessary to touch more than the bed covers. Each said what he thought of the illness of the said Lord and in conclusion, considered it deplorable. I told them that with his youth there still was some hope and that God and Nature sometimes do things that to Physicians and Surgeons seem impossible.

My consultation was . . . (here a long discussion is omitted; it can be found in any reprint of the "Apology and Treatise" if desired—ED.)

My discourse was well approved by the Physicians and Surgeons.

The consultation finished, we went to the patient and made three openings in the thigh, draining a great quantity of pus and serum and at the same time I removed several little bony spicules. I did not want to drain too much of the serum for fear of depleting his strength. Two or three hours later I had them make a bed near his with clean, white sheets. Then a strong man put him in it and he was very happy to be taken out of his dirty, stinking bed. Soon after he asked to sleep, which he did for four hours, when everyone in the house began to rejoice, especially his brother, the Duc d'Ascot.

In the following days I made injections into the depths

of the ulcer cavities with Egyptiac dissolved sometimes in brandy and at others in wine. To cleanse and dry the soft spongy flesh I applied compresses to the bottoms of the sinuses and hollow tents of lead, always for the purpose of providing drainage of the serum, over which I applied a great plaster of diachalcitheos dissolved in wine. Also I bandaged it so dextrously he had no pain. Thus soothed, the fever promptly began to diminish. Then I had him drink wine diluted moderately with water, knowing it restores and quickens the spirits. And all the things we agreed on in the conference were accomplished in proper time and order. And as his pain and fever receded, he began always to feel better. He let two of his Surgeons and a Physician go, so there were only three with him.

(Paré goes on to describe the honor paid him by the citizens of Heinaut in gratitude for his care of their beloved Marquis. He visited other Belgian cities including Antwerp and Bruxelles and finally was escorted back to his house in Paris by the Marquis' Steward and two pages. See also pg. 64—ED.)

Gunshot Through the Hand   (MIII,732)

I know nothing worth remembering (from the trip to Bourges, 1562—ED.) except one of the boys of the King's private kitchen who approached the city wall before it was surrendered, crying in a loud voice, "Huguenot,[141] Huguenot, shoot here, shoot here!" Having his arm upraised and his hand extended, a soldier shot a bullet through his hand. Having received the wound, he came to find me to dress it. M. le Connestable, seeing the boy with

---

[141] Huguenot—the name given the French Protestants; the origin of the word is unknown.

his hand all bloody and in tears, demanded who wounded him. Then a Gentleman who saw the shot, told him it was well done, since he cried, "Huguenot, shoot here, shoot here." Then the Connestable said the Huguenot was a good marksman and had a kind heart, since he could as well have shot him through the head, which he might have done easier than in the hand. I dressed the said cook, who was quite sick. He recovered, but with weakness of the hand and his companions have since called him 'Huguenot'; he is still living.

Gunshot of Spine; Paraplegia   (MIII,733)

The King commanded me, at the request of Madame la Connestable to go to her house and to treat M. le Connestable, who got a pistol shot in the middle of the dorsal spine (at the battle of St. Denis, November 10, 1567—ED.). He lost all feeling and movement of his thighs and legs; his excrements were retained, he could not pass urine and nothing by stool, because the spinal medulla, from which spring the nerves (to carry feeling and movement to the lower parts) were broken, torn and lacerated by the vehemence of the bullet. He also lost his understanding and reason and in a few days he died.

Wormy Abscess of Throat. Ranula with Stones   (MIII,733)

I treated a Spanish Gentleman (at Bayonne, 1565—ED.) who had a great, enormous abscess of the throat. He came to have himself touched by the late King Charles for scrofula. I opened his abscess where there was found a great quantity of creeping worms, as large as the point of a bobbin, having black heads. And it had a great quantity of rotten flesh.

Moreover, he had under his tongue a swelling called Ranula, which hindered him uttering his words and to eat and swallow his food. He prayed me with clasped hands to open it for him if it could be done without peril to his person. This I did promptly and found under my lancet a solid body, which was five stones like those one draws from the bladder. The largest was the size of a little almond and the others like little long beans, being five in number. In this swelling was more than four silver teaspoonsful of a glairy, yellow fluid. I left him in the hands of a Surgeon of the town to complete his cure.

Plague—Persistent Epistaxis (MIII,734)

M. le Fontaine, Chevalier of the Order of the King, had a high, continuous, pestilent fever accompanied by many carbuncles in different parts of the body. For two days he bled from the nose and none could stanch it. From this flux the fever ceased, with a profuse sweat. Soon after the carbuncles suppurated. He was dressed by me and cured by the Grace of God. (See also pg. 138—ED.)

Bibliography

Material Sources and Interesting Collateral Reading

1. Batiffol, L.: *The Century of the Renaissance*. London, Wm. Heinemann, Ltd., 1916.
2. de Laruelle, L. and Sendrail, M.: *Textes Choisis de Ambroise Paré*. Paris, Soc. les Belles Lettres, 1953.
3. Doe, Janet: *A Bibliography of the Works of Ambroise Paré, etc.* Chicago, University of Chicago Press, 1937.
4. Johnson, Tho.: *The Works of That Famous Chirurgien Ambroise Parey, Translated out of the Latin, etc.* London, E:C:, 1665.
5. Keynes, Geoffrey: *The Apologie and Treatise of Ambroise Paré, etc.* Chicago, University of Chicago Press, 1952.
6. La Paulmier, Stephen: *Ambroise Paré, d'après de Nouveux Documents, etc.* Paris, Perrin et Cie., 1887.
7. Malgaigne, J. F.: *Oeuvres Complètes d'Ambroise Paré*. Paris, J. B. Bailliere, 1840.
8. Michelin: *Les Guides Régionaux* (several). Paris, Services de Tourisme Michelin, 1957.
9. Packard, F. P.: *Life and Times of Ambroise Paré*. New York, Paul C. Hoeber, Inc., 1926.
10. Paget, Stephen: *Ambroise Paré and His Times, 1510-1590*. New York and London, G. P. Putnam's Sons, 1897.
11. Wickersheimer, C. A.: *La Médicine et les Médicines en France a l'Époque de la Renaissance*. Paris, A. Maloine, Ed., 1906.

Index

(Asterisks indicate members of the healing arts. Italic numerals locate explanatory footnotes.)

*Vesalius, 7
*Viart, Claude, *100*, 107, 114, 119, 146, 156, 158, 161
*de Vieux, Antoine, 105
*de Vigo, Jean, 57, 66, 162
Villaine Castle, *68*, 162
de Villars, Marquis, 78
Vinegar for hemostasis, 67
*de Violaines, Dr. Olivier, *11*, 19, 31, 102, 105, 114
Viper bite, 129
Vitré, 116
Vive(r), sting of, 132, 133
Vocal cord paralysis, 45
Voiding, delayed, effect, 92
Vomited worms, 115

Vomiting, therapeutic, 125, 154
Voyages in Divers Places, 156
Vulva, pruritis, 107

W

Wen, removal, 11
Witches, 123, 124
Wizards, 124
Wooden leg, 158, 159, 160, 169
Worms
  abscess, 190
  osteomyelitis skull, 24
  intestinal, 128
  teeth, 90
  vomited, 115
Wrestler, death of, 163